The recipes and techniques recommended for use with medical grade essential oils. Young Living Essential Oils are the only oils I feel comfortable with consistently recommending for use in animals. Use of other brands of oils may prove dangerous to certain animals.

Crow River Animal Hospital & Dental Clinic
1969 County Road 5 SW
Howard Lake, MN 55349
Phone: 320-286-3277
www.CrowRiverAnimalHospital.com
CrowRiverAnimalHospital@gmail.com

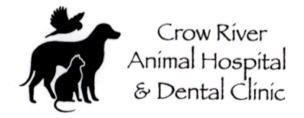

Copyright 2011

Table of Contents

About the Author..................5

Preface..................6
Disclosure..................14
Acknowledgements..................15
Vet to Vet..................16
Vet to Distributor..................20
Essential Oils – The Basics..................22
    What are Essential Oils?..................22
    Citrus Oils..................23
    Absolutes..................24
    Wild Crafted vs. Organic Essential Oils..................24
Distillation of Essential Oils..................26
    How Are Herbs and Oils Different?..................29
    What is Therapeutic Grade?..................30
    Four Main Ways to Use Oils..................30
Models of Aromatherapy..................31
The Basics of Using Oils in Animals..................33
    Common Misconceptions..................33
Essential Oils for Cats..................41
    NingXia Red..................43
    Car Rides..................44
    Hairballs..................44
    Litteroma..................45
    Respiratory Conditions..................49
    Abscesses..................51
    Kitty Raindrop Technique (KRDT)..................55
    Ear Mites..................60

- Feline Leukemia...62

DOGS...64
- Arthritis...65
- Incontinence (Urinary)......................................71
- Ear Infections...73
- Cruciate Injuries (Knee Injury).........................76
- Allergies...80
- Hot Spots...82
- Kennel Cough..85
- Diarrhea...87

HORSES..89

- Colic..90
- Laminitis (aka Founder)....................................92
- Strangles..94
- Thrush..100
- Navicular Disease (Syndrome).......................102
- White Line Disease (Seedy Toe)....................104
- Rain Rot...106
- Raindrop Technique for Horses.....................107
- Vitaflex..116

Supplements and Dosing Suggestions.....124
- BLM Capsules..124
- Detoxzyme...125
- Digest + Cleanse..125
- Inner Defense..126
- Juva Cleanse..126
- K & B Tincture..127
- Life 5..127
- Longevity...128
- Omega Blue...129

ParaFree..129

PD 80/20..130

Rehemogen..130

Sulfurzyme..131

NingXia Red...132

Whole Food Supplements..........................134

The information in this book is not intended to diagnose, prescribe or treat any medical illness or condition. If an animal or human you know has a health concern, I encourage you to seek the advice of a qualified health care professional.

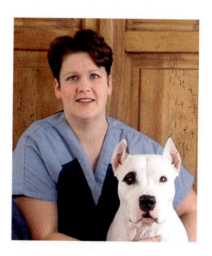

About the Author

Melissa Shelton DVM graduated in 1999 from the University of Minnesota, College of Veterinary Medicine. From childhood, Dr. Shelton knew she wanted to become a veterinarian. A love of nature and animals propelled her dream into a reality. Within veterinary college, Dr. Shelton received very traditional training toward her veterinary career – focused on the fundamentals of veterinary medicine. Additionally, she pursued training and participated in directed studies in avian orthopedics and in avian and exotic animal medicine and surgery.

Beyond veterinary college, Dr. Shelton has focused additional and extensive training in small animal dentistry, whole foods nutrition, holistic veterinary medicine, and especially in the chemistry and science behind the medical use of essential oils. Dr. Shelton strives to provide the veterinary community with the scientific data necessary for all animals to benefit from true therapeutic and medical grade essential oils.

Preface

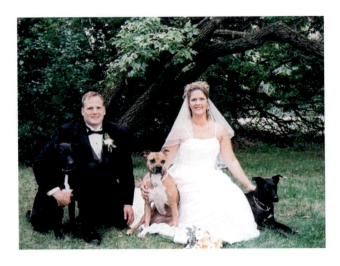

It was the year 2001. I had graduated from veterinary school in 1999, was newly engaged to my high school sweetheart Winston, and was ready to begin a new life and career. As my wedding date approached, there was a problem. My husband-to-be had warts all over his hands, and being a typical bride, I wanted beautiful pictures of our hands showing our new wedding rings. Horrible, ugly warts did not fit into this plan. We had done everything that traditional medicine offered. We had cut off the warts, frozen off the warts, painted on medicines, and even applied duct tape to the warts. Nothing had worked and we were running out of time. Our minister recommended that we try using the essential oil of clove to get rid of the warts. Thankfully, she recommended using Young Living Essential Oils, and with these truly therapeutic grade oils we saw results. Within 3 months, his hands were completely clear of warts and our wedding pictures were gorgeous.

One would think that this experience would have propelled me into using essential oils on a regular basis, but it did not. The clove oil was placed into a cabinet, and sat there for another 7 years. We were young and healthy and had no children at that point. Our motivation for natural and powerful remedies was not a priority in my life or career. As a new graduate of veterinary school, it felt as if I knew it all. I had all of this great new knowledge – and could fix any case that came my way. Of course, life teaches otherwise. As time went on, veterinary cases for which I had no answers began to frustrate me. Even though I was continually learning and seeking out new information, and had begun to incorporate other holistic healing modalities into my practice, there were still those frustrating cases for which there appeared to be no answers.

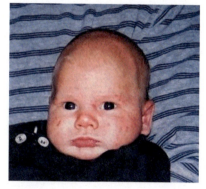

But, it would be my own family that would drive me back into the realm of essential oils. In 2002, we were blessed with our daughter Ramie. My husband Winston is challenged with a Tourette's-like syndrome, as well as his father, his brother, and my own brother. When Ramie was 2 ½ years old, we recognized that she too, was developing some tics. Then in 2005, our son Reiker was born.

When my son was a newborn baby, we noticed what we were told were "normal" skin issues. "Classic" cradle cap, baby eczema, and baby acne were conditions described by everyone who saw our son. However, when he was a few months old, he developed the coordination to scratch at his own head. Unfortunately, this showed us that his skin was in fact itching, and he would scratch until the skin was damaged and bloody. No longer were we dealing with skin that just looked bad. We would be up all night with our little baby, having him wear mittens, hats – you name it – trying to keep him from destroying his delicate skin. It was terribly stressful, resulting in many sleepless nights and tears.

As a veterinarian – I knew that this was NOT normal. I was never really comfortable with him having the other "normal" skin conditions either, as it didn't really make sense to me to have a fresh perfect new baby, have skin problems. With our new found horror of his itching, I had to find answers. We went to pediatricians, allergy specialists, naturopaths, homeopaths, chiropractors, kinesiologists, shamans, and Reiki Masters – I wanted to find someone with an answer – but alas, no one did.

I started to look at the situation as I would for a dog. I had started to notice a direct correlation with breast feeding and the itching. However, I was assured that he had tested negative for all food allergies by the traditional allergist, and even the kinesiologist could not find a direct correlation with diet and the reaction. So, I did what I would do for any pet in my hospital – A DIET TRIAL. Since he was breast feeding, it was really a diet trial for me. My diet consisted of eating only plain chicken and water for 2 weeks. And, low and behold, my son was normal. I had my answer. He was definitely reacting to something I was eating, and it was passing through my breast milk and causing an allergic reaction in him.

Next, I introduced foods one at a time to see where the reaction would rear its ugly head. I kept a very exact diet log documenting everything I ate or drank, what time I ate or drank it, when our son was breast fed, and if he had a reaction to the feeding. After a while, it became incredibly confusing to figure out which items were causing the problem. He would react when I had eaten yogurt, but not to milk. He would react if I had ketchup on a hamburger patty, but not to chili with hamburger and tomatoes. He even seemed to react to me having a soft drink! Every time I thought I found an answer – dairy, tomatoes, beef, citrus... something else would prove that to be wrong. I didn't give up though. I had 2 weeks of diet logs and poured over them to find the answer.

Thankfully, a friend of mine came over and was telling me of her "disgust" of corn syrup. It was in so many foods, was certainly causing health problems, and it was almost impossible to buy anything that didn't contain it. LIGHT BULB!!! I grabbed my diet log – and guess what. Corn syrup was in every item that my son reacted to. Yogurt sweetened with corn syrup, white bread sweetened with corn syrup, ketchup sweetened with corn syrup! However, I was assured by multiple medical doctors that there was no way that a baby could react to corn syrup, and especially not through the mother's breast milk. Tell that to my 4 month old son, scratching his face and head until it bled!

Corn syrup is in almost every commercial food item today. Bread, soda, popsicles and freezies, ice cream, yogurt, fruit snacks, canned fruits, ketchup, hot chocolate mix, crackers, graham crackers, cereals, chocolate milk, tomato soup, hot dogs, lunch meat; the list goes on and on.

We drastically changed our whole family's diet for our son. We faithfully read ingredient labels and purchased only wholesome foods that did not contain corn syrup, high fructose corn syrup, corn syrup solids or anything else related to corn syrup. We saw amazing changes, and my son was normal again. We hadn't realized that he was also having quite a bit of digestive problems, which also disappeared with the new changes.

However, as we changed all of this – we noted something else. My husband and my 4 year old daughter – improved significantly in THEIR tics and symptoms. More importantly, we found another amazing correlation. When we would have a "dietary break" – and they would eat something with corn syrup or chemicals in it – their symptoms would escalate, usually within 24 hours.

Of course, once you clean up your diet – it becomes easier and easier to recognize items that cause a problem. What I have found for our family – has encouraged me to teach others what diet can do for their health concerns. As more and more people eliminate corn syrup, food dyes, artificial sweeteners, preservatives, MSG, and other food chemicals – the results are remarkable. Children that had their diets changed did not need medications or needed much less of them. Adults found that they were having much less skin problems, such as eczema. Children's behavior in general (even in children that didn't have behavioral challenges) – seemed much more easy going and pleasant.

Over and over again, there were significant improvements for children and adults when corn syrup and chemicals were removed from their life. Conditions including Attention Deficit Disorder (ADD), Attention Deficit Hyperactive Disorder (ADHD),

Tourette's syndrome, Asperger's, Obsessive Compulsive Disorder (OCD), Anxiety disorders, Autism, Pediatric Autoimmune Neuropsychiatric Disorders Associated with Streptococcal Infections (PANDA's), and multiple other behavioral and neurologic issues; all had major connections with what we were putting into our bodies.

So what does this have to do with my journey towards using essential oils? This whole experience opened my eyes to the fact that a seemingly small thing, can indeed matter. Something as small and supposedly unimportant as corn syrup or a food chemical, *can* cause incredibly profound "side effects" in life and health.

However, I believe that small things can also enact life changing good as well.

As I was starting to comprehend the consequences that un-natural chemicals could bring into our human lives, we were starting to acknowledge some very interesting cases in our veterinary hospital. We encountered dogs that would become very ill when household odor-eliminating sprays were used. We documented cats with elevated liver enzymes from eating on kitchen counters cleaned with a certain polishing compound. We witnessed chronic ear infections and allergies completely disappear when households changed to all natural cleaning products. Use of air fresheners, fabric softeners, and perfumes now appeared on the differential list as a contributor to frustrating chronic illnesses. The horrible effects of everyday household toxins were showing up everywhere – once you knew to look for them.

In good consciousness, I could no longer use these products in my veterinary hospital. If these products were harmful for the animals in my care – what were they doing to my family? I threw out all of my air fresheners, plug in devices, and sprays. Odor control became an issue, as my veterinary hospital is within my home. I felt rather stuck – but I would rather have bad odors than hurt an animal or my loved ones.

We had already started to look toward natural medicines and a holistic approach to life and health for our family. My children's challenges demanded it. As part of this exploration, I attended a class through our local community education program. The class was on natural remedies for all sorts of things; from colds and flu to ADD/ADHD. When I walked into the class, there was a wonderful smell coming from a diffuser. I had found my answer for natural health care for my family, and I was transported back to Young Living Essential Oils once again. But, could the essential oils be safely used for odor control in my vet clinic? The instructor of the class said she knew of many people using Young Living Oils on animals, but of course, I am not one to take one person's word for it. I have to research everything for myself.

I bought every book on essential oils that I could, reading them cover to cover in days. I attended every local class on essential oils that was offered. Inevitably at these classes, people would find out that I was a veterinarian, and they would proceed to share all of their stories on how the oils had been used to treat their dog or cat, horse or goat. I was intrigued. Then as my research and learning turned to my veterinary community – I received a completely different response. DANGER, DANGER, DANGER...Do NOT use essential oils in pets, and don't even diffuse them around cats. Here were the top names in holistic veterinary medicine, and they were largely against the use of essential oils. How could it be that hundreds and thousands of Young Living members were using their oils safely on their pets, but in general the veterinary community believed that essential oils could be very harmful and recommended avoiding them?

I am not one to allow a mystery to go unsolved. My trek continued, and I was determined to find out the truth about oils and animals. Obviously, I would have to do the research and gather the proof myself. I had already been using Young Living oils for my human family for some time. I was diffusing in almost every room of my own home, and my cats seemed actually drawn to the rooms with diffusers in them. Kittens were born in rooms with diffusers running, and cats routinely slept inside my case of essential oils – they loved the oils. People commented on how intelligent our kittens were, how they looked into the eyes of humans, and how they seemed so much older than they actually were.

I started using oils directly on my own cats, dogs, horses, chickens, and cow. After all, if I did not believe I could use the oils for my own animals, why should I ever recommend them for a patient? All of my animals get routine blood and urine tests, so they were a great model for monitoring against any potential side effects from essential oils. With over 10 animals being exposed to essential oils almost 24 hours a day through diffusion, topical application, and ingestion – there was a definite ability to document their health and responses to essential oils.

Then in my veterinary hospital, patients presented that were close to euthanasia or for which I had no answers to offer traditionally – I now began offering essential oil therapies. This is where I started. In the hopeless cases, that had nothing to lose. I was coming up with the same amazing results that so many pet owners had already communicated to me. There were situations where traditional medicine offered NOTHING – and I was getting responses to essential oils.

The cases with the animals in my practice and Young Living Essential Oils, were nothing less than amazing. Although it may seem like a fast progression, to go from novice essential oil user, to being known internationally in veterinary aromatherapy in under 2 years…you would just have to know me. I never do anything "lightly". Considering that Veterinary College is only 4 years, and covers every subject in medicine and surgery – 2 years of intense study and medical use of essential oils in animals is really very significant. I throw myself into everything I do, and essential oils had immediately become a passion for me. I condensed 10+ years of essential oil education and experience, into a 1 year adventure. I have lost count of how many essential oil books I own – and I have read each one, cover to cover. I have listened to almost every CD and recorded educational call that is available – and I don't just listen to them, I memorize them. I have purchased every reference I could find about oils and animals, and I feel proud of the fact that I have found books that even my teachers did not know about.
But with all of the classroom learning and book smarts – nothing compares to actually using essential oils to treat animals. On our 15 acre farm, I currently have around 20 rescued cats, 13 pet cats, 5 dogs, 3 horses, 1 pony, 1 cow, 1 goat, and over 20 chickens. My

wonderful collection of strays, misfits, injured and ill animals – allow me a great opportunity to "play with the oils". Many of the animals that we took on were hopeless cases. They had no options in life, except to be adopted by a vet, who would go to extraordinary measures to try to make them comfortable and to try to save their lives.

We are now fortunate enough to have clients demanding treatments with essential oils in our practice. Every single case in our hospital benefits from the use of essential oils, even if it is only from basic diffusing. By using oils every day in our veterinary clinic, I have been blessed with an amazing opportunity to witness the powerful effects of truly therapeutic essential oils.

It has always been a passion of mine to educate and share what I have learned; from which diets work the best for my clients to which suture material pit bulls tolerate. I am fortunate that essential oils are combining all of my passions into one; healing animals, teaching, and writing. I hope that you enjoy this book, as much as I have enjoyed creating it.

May you and your family (furry and otherwise) benefit as our family has.

Melissa Shelton DVM

Disclosure

I feel it is an important aspect to let you know that I *am* a distributor for Young Living Essential Oils. However, as a veterinarian, I am basically a distributor for EVERY product that I carry or sell. To me, this makes no difference in my recommendations of which products to use. Yes, Young Living has a "multi-level marketing" component to it, and yes, some people have chosen the annoying "sales person" route to sell the products. However, I see this with my traditional veterinary products as well. Some companies have wonderful sales reps that I love, and others make me want to hide when they come calling.

The world is full of sales. I sell my veterinary services and products for a profit, and would not be in business if I didn't. Products and services I choose to sell are carefully considered. If I recommend a product only for a profit – then I would not be a successful veterinarian for very long!

The products I recommend must work for my patients, or else my patients would not be coming to me. So whether I pick a traditional therapy, or an alternative therapy – the bottom line is that it must be safe and must get results. What I recommend is not about a paycheck, it is about what is effective.

Acknowledgements

I would first like to begin by thanking D. Gary Young for his commitment to creating the world's best essential oils – with only the highest of therapeutic qualities. Without this dedication, none of the miracles that I have witnessed would have occurred. By sharing his knowledge on essential oils, he educated those who initially taught me how to use essential oils. Gary has withstood countless criticisms and hardships from "mainstream" healthcare, and yet has remained dedicated to the wondrous powers that essential oils hold for our health. For that, I commend and thank him.

Next, I would like to thank Angela and Mark Meredith for their community education class that started it all. I couldn't have been more fortunate to "fall" into a society of essential oil users who are so devoted to education. The tremendous support that I have received from them, is unmatched.

I also wish to thank Cherie Ross and her entire organization. Cherie teaches so many classes, and truly dedicates her life to helping others. She is passionate about saving lives, and has seen and participated in many miracles in her "career" using Young Living Essential Oils. Without her vast knowledge and experience, I would have never learned what I needed to know to start utilizing oils medically.

Finally, it is important to recognize the importance of Young Living members. What a vast resource to have this incredible community of people, who share a common passion and mission. The majority of the members, share their lives and oils with animals, thereby contributing greatly to the data that can be pooled together to show the safety and efficacy of Young Living oils to the veterinary world.

Vet to Vet

When I first started using essential oils it was for my human family. Naturally, if there was a product I was going to use on my children, I wanted to learn more about it. So I sought out classes and books on the topic. Of course, as most veterinarians can sympathize – as soon as other people attending these classes found out that I was a veterinarian, they told me stories upon stories about their pets. The interesting thing became that because we were at a class for essential oil use, most of their stories involved the use of essential oils on their pets.

I had a very critical eye at first. Obviously, a dog or cat that got better from the owner using essential oils – could have just gotten better on its own. However, I had to remind myself that sometimes when I give an antibiotic for frequent urination – it too may get better on its own, having nothing to do with an actual bladder infection. In medicine, we tend to pat ourselves on the back when a pet gets better. I can't express how lucky I was to have one of the pioneers of veterinary thinking right in my veterinary college. Dr. Carl Osborne from the University of Minnesota, College of Veterinary Medicine is a strong name in veterinary research, especially urology. Although we may have thought it corny at the time, he taught us classes on the basic philosophy of practicing traditional veterinary medicine. Topics within his lectures were *How to avoid the 'energy vampire'*, *How to take care of yourself and your patients*, as well as *How to evaluate your patients with problem and evidence based medicine*. One phrase I remember him saying is "Sometimes the patient gets better, despite of anything that we have done."

I think that it is also true to say, that sometimes a patient does get better because of something we have done. But, it also has to be said that sometimes a patient gets better because of something an owner has done. I have been in that boat before. An owner comes up with some strange treatment for their pet that they found on the internet – and now this becomes the miracle cure that saved their dog – not the week long hospital stay with IV fluids, IV medications, or around the clock care. However, I would be naive and wrong to not acknowledge that an owner has sometimes found a home remedy that was actually very helpful to their pet. We would be ignorant to think that just as we are veterinarians, that we have all of the answers.

This can certainly be the feeling with essential oils. I have told my clients not to use essential oils in the past. I didn't understand them, had heard tales of toxicity, and felt that it was best to err on the side of caution. But, I have learned that when we do not know about a non-traditional remedy – it may be best to say "I do not have enough knowledge in that area – and cannot give you a proper opinion on it."

I think it is still important to document and work with owners who want to use a non-traditional treatment for their animal. Alienating the client is certainly no way to help our patient, and will result in our inability to learn anything new. Certainly we can discuss the fact that we are concerned with safety issues not being documented…however, I try to remember that when a certain popular Non-Steroidal Anti-inflammatory Drug (NSAID) came onto the veterinary market, we all jumped to use it. However, within months we started to see some cases of horrible side effects. However, we did not condemn the product. We learned how to better use it and performed blood tests to screen and monitor patients – but right or wrong, the veterinary community continued to dispense this potentially dangerous drug. In many patients the benefits outweighed the risks of using the drug. Severely arthritic dogs were likely to be put to sleep when their quality of life was declining, so if the NSAID gave them relief, their life was saved. They could either die from the symptoms of a treatable disease, or potentially die from side effects of a drug that relieved those symptoms. Six of one, half a dozen of another.

The important element that I have found with the use of essential oils in animals – is truly related to the quality of the essential oil. Although there are likely to be companies other than Young Living that have therapeutic grades of essential oils, I have not found them to be consistent. If every other batch of Amoxicillin you ordered for your veterinary hospital carried side effects or lack of efficacy – how long would you want to carry that product? I feel that essential oils much mirror the use of Flea and Tick Preventives in the traditional veterinary world. Most would agree that veterinarians have seen vast differences in efficacy and safety when comparing veterinary brands to over-the-counter products. I have witnessed cats seizure and even die from flea products labeled for use in cats – purchased at chain discount stores. Why should essential oils be any different? Grades in quality do exist. Unfortunately, I have found that veterinarians have been reluctant to focus on the fact that it may truly be differences in the quality of an essential oil that are causing the reported adverse reactions in pets.

Every report of toxicity that I have researched – either has incomplete information, is poorly documented, or is purely hearsay. The more complete reports that I can find, outline products that seem poorly formulated, by those who are jumping on the band wagon to create a natural pet product for sale. Guaranteed, these people mainly know nothing about true medical uses of essential oils or of the grades and qualities of oils, and certainly have no veterinary degree. When business is the motivation, the cheapest supply of essential oils will be sought after. These are generally the perfume grade oils that are not suitable for use in animals - ever.

In my own life, I have become so cautious that I avoid natural cleaners that contain essential oils of unknown quality. I would much rather purchase an unscented cleaner, and add my own essential oils to it if desired. This may sound extreme, but to me – the risk of using a poor grade essential oil around my animals and children seems just as bad as the toxic chemicals contained in regular household cleaners.

Omitting the usage of truly medical grade oils from my life – is not something I am willing to do. They have become such an amazing part of treating pets – that to exclude them from my arsenal – would be like removing an entire class of treatment from my use. Imagine saying – I will never do surgery again in my clinic – how many pets would suffer? Well, I find the same "class of treatment" in essential oils. There would be a huge hole in my practice if I were unable to use this modality any longer.

Now, for some it is necessary to get over the fact that Young Living has a business component to it. However, I remind you that so does every other market that we bring into our vet clinic. Every item we sell is marked up, or it should be if you plan on staying in business. Making money off of the products and services we sell is necessary if you would like to make a living and keep practicing. Certainly there are many "multi-level marketing" companies out there with a less than stellar reputation. But, I urge you to not condemn every product based on this experience. Use common sense and experience things for yourself before you decide. There have certainly been many traditional veterinary products released with promises of greatness, that end up being a total failure or actually even harmful to animals. However, veterinarians often keep purchasing items from that company! Why the double standard? I don't really know. But, I urge you to keep an open mind and do not miss out on an opportunity for great healing, due to human obstinance.

All natural remedies seem to find themselves in a position of having to prove themselves. If they did not result in a miracle or have some amazing response, we rack it up to the fact that natural remedies must not work. But, how many traditional cases in the veterinary hospital have not responded completely to the first prescription, needed a repeat round of treatment, or just perplex us. We generally don't denounce all antibiotics if our first choice didn't clear up a bladder infection. We just reason that we picked the wrong antibiotic, have a resistant bacterial strain, or mis-diagnosed a bladder infection.

Please look at essential oils in this manner. Remember that every time you wish to use them – you need to think of them like any other veterinary treatment. You must have a good quality, it must be used properly, and monitoring may be desired. Essential oils are not the be all and end all of natural remedies, and do not replace every medical therapy. However, in my experience, they have powerful abilities, that should not be overlooked.

Vet to Distributor

I am routinely asked, "How do I get my vet involved with Essential Oils?" Unfortunately, my answer is "You don't." I am very realistic in the fact that veterinarians do not want to be *sold* a product or a new treatment. What often draws a veterinarian to a new modality, are the responses they see. As I meet other veterinarians using essential oils, they often have started using essential oils in their human life, long before they ever used them in their profession. Approaching a vet with a business opportunity to use essential oils will likely meet you with a total shut down. Sharing your personal experiences with essential oils, sharing oils with the vet so that they can "feel" the results, and working hand-in-hand with them when your animals are using oils are the best ways to gain their interest. Fortunately, the tides are starting to turn, and holistic veterinarians everywhere are starting to seek out information about different treatments, including essential oils. Nevertheless, most veterinarians would still like to be advised on how to use this treatment from a fellow veterinarian.

My greatest advice for those who would like to introduce essential oils into animal markets - whether they are groomers, shelters, training facilities, horse farms, boarding kennels, or veterinary clinics – is to first introduce odor controlling methods for the facility. See the chapter "You Never Get a Second Chance to Make a First Impression". Odor control is certainly something that all animal facilities need to consider. And offering a safe, effective, and pleasant option to this dilemma can be a rewarding situation for all involved. Many times, I have seen people start with "Aromatherapy" for odor control only – and they magically start to see the "other" benefits in the animals around them. From less anxiety, to less illness – it is quickly realized that there is much more to Aromatherapy than "smelling good".

For those facilities hoping to provide more with essential oils – the sky is the limit! I have great fun brainstorming on how animal related facilities could use essential oils in their business. How wonderful would it be if your boarding facility offered to diffuse Peace and Calming for your dog if they became nervous? Would you love it if your dog groomer offered bathing with all natural non-toxic shampoo? What if the groomer could add additional essential oils into a shampooing that would help with arthritis discomfort or other concerns – would you be interested? I know I would!

My hope is that this book can help to bridge that avenue of communication between you and your veterinarian, or any other animal related provider. Having a reference written by a veterinarian will hopefully help everyone in their quest to use essential oils for their Natural Pet Care.

Essential Oils – The Basics

There is so much wonderful and complete information available on the chemistry and properties of essential oils. Repeating what has already been written would not be a good use of this book. I urge you to read and reference the following books for a better understanding of essential oils. There you will find the medical properties, chemical constituents, and historical uses for each essential oil. If you only have one book to invest in, I recommend starting with the Essential Oils Desk Reference.

Essential Oils Desk Reference – Essential Science Publishing
The Chemistry of Essential Oils Made Simple – David Stewart Ph.D., D.N.M.
Essential Oils: Integrative Medical Guide – D. Gary Young, ND
Reference Guide for Essential Oils – Connie and Alan Higley

What are Essential Oils?

An essential oil is the volatile, fat-soluble portion of the fluids from a plant. They contain the aromatic (fragrant) compounds of that plant. Many parts of a plant can be distilled to obtain the essential oil; flowers, fruit, seeds, leaves, stems, branches, and/or roots.

Essential oils are the life blood of the plant, "essential" to the life processes of the plant (bacterial, fungal, and viral defense as well as healing). If you remove the essential oil from the plant, the plant dies. The essential oil acts much like the blood within our body. Our blood purifies, protects, and acts as a defense in our body – as does the essential oil in the plant.

These oils can perform the same functions for our body as they do for a plant; aid in health and healing, protect from bacteria, fungi, and viruses, regulate plant functions acting as hormones and ligands, promote homeostasis in an organism, attack harmful bacteria and leave the good bacteria, as well as protect the plant from sunlight, excessive heat, and dehydration. When a plant is injured it weeps essential oils to promote healing and protect from infection. Essential oils can do the same activity for our cells at the site of an injury.

Intelligence comes from Mother Nature – oils do not want to destroy the plant, just like blood should not destroy our body. Oils need to protect their host from harmful invaders – so they can be aggressive when needed. In our body, our white blood cells do not destroy our own cells unless it is needed – and unless we are toxic and malfunctioning, our bodies have the intelligence to do things properly – so do essential oils.

Essential Oils are not like fatty oils, vegetable oils, or fatty acids such as olive oil, flax oil, fish oils, etc… Fatty oils are pressed from the seeds of a plant. Fatty oils are not essential to the life of a plant; they are used for storage of energy for the seed to grow. Although essential oils are fat soluble, they do not moisturize and shouldn't feel greasy by themselves.

Essential oils contain hundreds of compounds, so complex that not ONE single oil has been completely analyzed for all of its ingredients scientifically. There are constituents in essential oils that have not yet been identified by science. AFNOR (Association Francaise de Normalization) only has minimum requirements to call an oil "that oil". So adulteration, cutting, and synthetic additives to make essential oils more affordable are rampant in the general market.

Citrus Oils

Citrus oils are considered essential oils but are produced by cold expression – pressing of the rinds. These oils are more likely to be adulterated or contaminated by pesticides, pollution, and other contaminants. So, trusted and clean sources for these oils are very important. Because these oils are from the rind, and encourage ripening of the fruit – furanoid compounds contained within these oils amplify ultraviolet light to accelerate the creation of sugars, and ripening of the fruit. From this same action, our skin can develop photosensitivity with citrus oils. If you apply photosensitizing oils to skin, and then expose that skin to intense sunlight, skin will often turn a strange grey coloration. Common single oils and oil blends to consider as photosensitive are Grapefruit, Lemon, Orange, Bergamot, Joy, Peace and Calming, White Angelica. Bergamot and Angelica Root are the two most photosensitizing oils. Joy blend contains high levels of Bergamot. 12-24 hours is generally enough time for the oil to be gone from the skin, with no risk of phototoxicity. The sun during the winter months (as we have in the Northern United States) is generally not as strong, and will not cause a reaction. Neither diffusion nor oral use of citrus oils will cause photosensitivity. During the summer months, it is well advised to put these oils "where the sun don't shine".

Grapefruit oil is different from Grapefruit meat or juice – if you are told not to ingest grapefruit with a prescription drug (statins for example), Grapefruit essential oil is okay for you to use and ingest.

Absolutes

Neroli, Jasmine, Vanilla, and Onycha are absolutes – and are not technically essential oils. Grain alcohol extraction is used to gather these essences. In general, absolutes should not be ingested or used orally. Onycha is used as tincture of benzoin in hospitals, even to this day, and has powerful antibacterial properties.

Wild Crafted vs. Organic Essential Oils

Where the plant matter comes from, how it is grown, and how it is harvested makes a huge difference in the quality of an essential oil. Wild crafted oils are often superior to organic oils. To be certified as organic in the United States, land only has to be chemical free for 3 years. Organic farmers often plant deep rooted plants, to help absorb and get rid of the chemicals in a previously non-organic field, as they know that the plant will leech the chemicals from the soil, helping them rid the soil of contamination. We can never know for sure when all of the previous chemicals used on a field will be absent from the plants and soil. Wild crafted generally should mean that the plants were obtained from "wild land". This often means that chemicals have never been used on the land. Finding a company that is dedicated to researching land history, studying wind patterns, and inspecting adjacent properties is rare. However, this is often what is necessary to make sure that chemicals are not contaminating their crops. Soils deficient in nutrients and minerals produce deficient plants. Deficient plants will produce deficient oils. However, the use of un-natural fertilizers will concentrate into a plant, thus passing into the essential oil. Even fertilizing with manure from livestock that were grazed on fields with herbicides, has been shown to inhibit plant growth. There are so many circumstances to consider in the production of an essential oil, you want to leave nothing to chance.

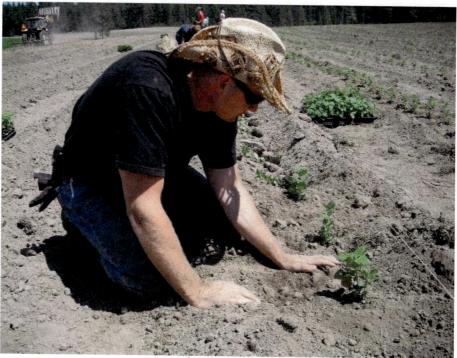

Planting Melissa

Distillation of Essential Oils

Distillation of plant matter for medical grade essential oils should be performed by steam only, and not with solvents. The distillation and collection chambers should be made of inert materials such as stainless steel and glass. The proper botanical genus, species, and cultivar should be used to collect the medical properties for that plant. When choosing an essential oil for a medical application, you often won't recognize what subspecies you should have unless you are trained. Lavender angustifolia and Lavendin oils are good examples of this. Lavendula angustifolia is the "heritage" form of lavender that still carries wonderful medicinal properties. Lavendin is a hybrid, only grown for fragrance and rapid growth, and would not be used for medical purposes. Many plants have subspecies; Ocotea, Copaiba, Helichrysum, even Peppermint – these subspecies can be very different, much like the varieties of apples are different from different trees. Finding a company that only picks the most medically active subspecies of the plants is important.

Environmental temperatures, water or drought conditions, time of day of harvest, how long a plant is "dried" prior to distillation, how it is handled, and the time, temperature, and pressure of distillation will all affect the constituents of the final oil produced. Every plant has an ideal method of distillation, and rigorous testing and attention to detail is important to discover the most optimal methods to obtain the most therapeutic and complete essential oil.

It takes 2000-3000 pounds of Melissa plants to create just 1 liter of essential oil. Sixteen pounds of peppermint plants are needed to make 1 ounce of peppermint essential oil. This is why the price between these two oils is so different. Poorer quality oil distillers use chemical solvents, make multiple passes (distill the plant material multiple times), and use high pressure to extract as much oil out of the plant as possible – only hoping to increase their yield and profits – but not having concern about the quality of this extorted oil.

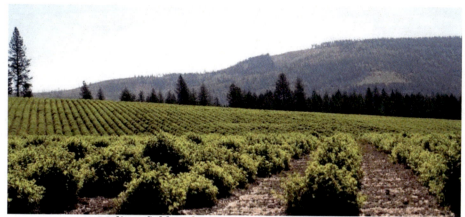
Melissa field at the Young Living Farm in Idaho

Medical grade distillers only collect oils from one pass, with low pressures and proper temperatures to ensure the perfect oil is extracted. Young Living tests every batch of oils multiple times, and with multiple labs. Oils are to be ideal in quality, or they are put back onto the land, as support for the next crop. Young Living grown oils that are "rejected" are NOT resold to others. Since Young Living cannot grow all of their own oils, they work with other growers to ensure the best possible quality. They inspect every farm, train the farmers and distillers, and are instrumental in every aspect of procuring medical grade oils. Even with this dedication, Young Living must occasionally reject a shipment of oils that do not meet medical standards – and unfortunately, those oils go back into the market. When using oils for medical purposes – there should be no question to the quality of the oil. Nova Vita is a human hospital based in Ecuador, where Young Living oils are even injected intravenously, into the bloodstream, of patients. For this application – the oils MUST be pure! This is the quality strived for in every oil produced by Young Living.

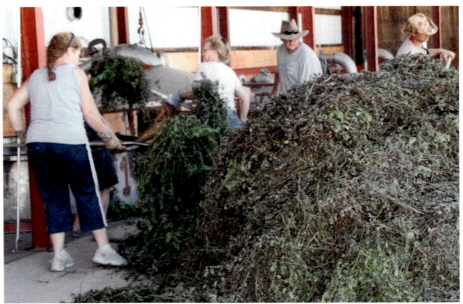
Thousands of pounds of Melissa being packed into the distiller.

It is very costly and time consuming to grow, farm, harvest, and distill correctly. Young Living is very dedicated to this – that is why they get good results – and create "oil snobs". It would be much cheaper to pay a laboratory technician to mix up chemicals, than it would be to run a complete farm and distillation practice. The scary part is that chemicals mixed up in a lab, can still be called "natural" if the chemical is found in nature.

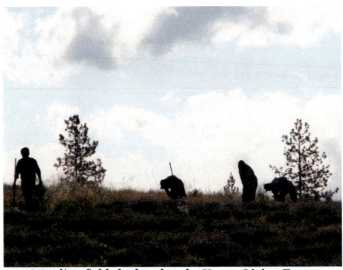
Weeding fields by hand at the Young Living Farm

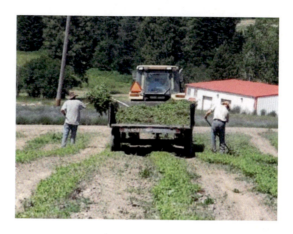

Therapeutic or medical grade oils have "life-force" within them – the vibrational energy of the plant is retained within a quality essential oil. Synthetic essential oils do not.

How Are Herbs and Oils Different?

Only small molecules (less than 300 atomic mass units) are distilled into essential oils. To utilize larger molecules from a plant – herbs are used. This is why herbs are still "good"; however they lack the essential oils which are lost in the drying process. One drop of peppermint essential oil equals the herb used to brew 26 cups of peppermint tea. There is no way that a pet or human could consume enough herbs to match the power that one drop of peppermint oil can contain. Herbs are rich in large particles, where essential oils are rich in small particles.

Herbs must also be ingested, digested, AND absorbed to be effective. We all know how hard it can be to make our animals take medications, but shoving multiple capsules of herbs down their throats can be quite impossible at times. Once we do get the herbs into the animal – then we still must rely on a competent digestive system to break down and absorb the nutrients. This is not always possible for a compromised animal to do properly. Sometimes we are trying to improve digestion and remedy digestive disorders – and asking the digestive system to "work" to absorb its remedy – is not always feasible. Essential oils can be absorbed transdermally (through the skin) and even inhaled to reach therapeutic levels. I cannot think of an easier way to administer therapeutic benefits to animals than that!

What is Therapeutic Grade?

Therapeutic grade, certified therapeutic grade, 100% natural, organic, wild-crafted...all of these "buzz" words are being thrown around in the aromatherapy world. Many companies are trying to cash in on the "therapeutic grade" hype of essential oils - and sell oils as therapeutic grade when there is much lacking in strength and purity. True therapeutic grade oils should have genus and species name of the plant on the bottle. They should also have supplement information – about ingestion of the oil – printed onto the label. This is an FDA requirement for dietary supplements – and proves that the oil can be taken orally. Truly therapeutic grade essential oils should also come in a dark bottle that is sealed until you open it. For me – I call the oils I use "medical grade" – as it distinguishes them above and beyond even "therapeutic grade".

Four Main Ways to Use Oils:

There are four main ways to absorb essential oils. Through the lungs, through the skin, within the gastrointestinal tract (by ingestion), and through absorbent tissues such as the mucus membranes in the rectum, vagina, or under the tongue. The fifth possible way of using essential oils is through hypodermic injection (generally into a tumor) or by intravenous administration by a physician only.

Models of Aromatherapy

There are three main models of Aromatherapy usage, and this is where much of the controversy can come in. Germans tend to use aromatherapy and essential oils through inhalation only. English and British schools of thought mainly use only VERY diluted essential oils in a massage application. The French model is what I have found to be most accurate when considering truly therapeutic grade (or medical grade) essential oil use. French aromatherapists will use oils topically (including neat), orally, and by inhalation.

Young Living members consist of 100's of thousands of people, who use the French model of aromatherapy everyday. To me, this is an enormous safety study in itself – for humans and for pets. Aromatherapy IS safe, when used with the proper oils. There has never been a death reported with essential oil use, except in the case of gross misuse. One woman was killed when she took huge amounts of Pennyroyal essential oil to cause an abortion. Another report was of an English baby who was killed by being given 4 grams of Wintergreen essential oil in one day!! This would be the equivalent of giving 9 bottles of aspirin! You still have to use essential oils responsibly. Certainly automobiles kill more people everyday than essential oils have EVER caused a serious health concern – however, the vast majority of us will still drive a car!

British models and thoughts of aromatherapy will scare you silly from oils. In general essential oils from England are of horrendous quality – so if you were using British oils, you *should* be cautious, overly dilute them, and only apply them topically. Veterinarians and Medical Doctors alike, will generally look for the worst thing that can happen with a "new" treatment – and will rest comfortably with the "danger diagnosis" – afraid of anything new. Even one book from a British author, is enough to make anyone leery of using ANY essential oil. Be cautious on which references you pick, many are inaccurate in regards to the use of truly medical grade oils.

Dr. David Stewart's book The Chemistry of Essential Oils Made Simple – has a wonderful section in Chapter One that fully explains all of the major essential oil books on the market – and which model of aromatherapy they are based on. This chapter has been a magnificent help for me when deciding on which books I wanted to invest in. Certainly to me, it was a huge waste of money to purchase a book that told me that I could not apply essential oils neat to the skin - of a human or an animal – when I already had been!

The Basics of Using Oils in Animals

Common Misconceptions:

There have been many things said about essential oils in animals. If they do not "want" them or they turn away from them – do not use them. Cats do not like Pine or Citrus oils. Valerian will build up in a system, and cannot be used. Grapefruit oil cannot be used while a human or pet is on medications. You can apply to the pads of animals; you shouldn't apply to the pads of animals. You need to part the fur or the oils won't be absorbed...

I have heard all of these statements, and many of them from people who have used essential oils for many, many years. I think that many times it is heard, believed, but never examined fully for the truth. Or it may be that the truth is just not out there to be found. I do know that I prefer to research all of the claims that I hear, as well as evaluate them from my experience and the experience of others.

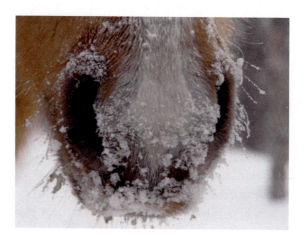

Pets are extremely sensitive to smell. If search and rescue dogs can trace the steps of a human, imagine how strong a plug-in air freshener must smell to them right at nose level! Along with this sensitive sniffer, also comes a physical sensitivity to artificial chemicals. We have documented some pretty interesting cases of liver and kidney value elevations from the use of cleaners, air fresheners, and odor eliminators. When a patient comes to us and smells of cigarette smoke, fabric softener, or perfume – I cringe. If I can smell these odors *on the pet*, imagine how strong the odors must be *in* that home. If you have ever gotten a headache after being exposed to someone's obnoxious perfume – just magnify this by 1000+ times – and you will be experiencing what a pet must experience.

Just because an odor is natural, does not mean it won't be offensive to a pet. We need to respect our pet's sense of smell when we use essential oils around them. Just like cats will start to run from you after getting pilled a few times, they may also need some treatments with natural remedies that will likewise make them flee the scene. There are unique circumstances where oils are needed medically, and we certainly deal with those as needed. But in everyday use of essential oils it is important to follow a few rules.

Always allow a pet an option to get away from an oil. When I diffuse an essential oil for the first time, I try to make sure it is in an open or larger room, and that any animals in my house, have the opportunity to leave the room if desired. I usually find that they actually gravitate toward the essential oil, but if need be, I want them to be able to get some fresh air. With birds in cages, just start out with a mild oil, and do not diffuse in a small, closed up room. Start farther away from animals that cannot leave the room, and stay with them the first few uses. Diffuse for all animals in small, short sessions first (15-20 minutes), and with a weak diffusing solution (2-4 drops in the ultrasonic diffuser). An ultrasonic water diffuser has endless combinations of diffusion strengths and times that you can vary. Gradually, over time, you can increase the duration of diffusion and the strength (how many drops of oil are added to the diffuser). In our home, we literally have a diffuser going 24 hours a day. Most of the time several diffusers. Our pets are exposed to essential oils 24 hours a day, they get routine blood work, and are examined by a veterinarian daily ☺ I have seen no ill effects, and only health benefits by their continued exposure to essential oils.

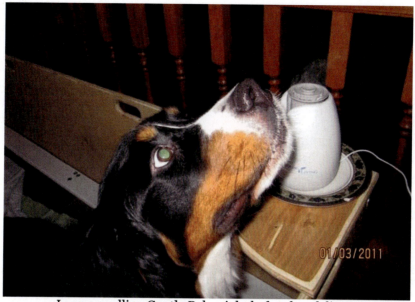
Logan smelling Gentle Baby right before her delivery

When applying oils to pets, generally more dilution is best at first. There are some oils and some circumstances where I apply oils "neat" or undiluted to an animal; however the safest rule of thumb is to dilute the oil with Young Living's V6 Oil Blend or with Extra Virgin Olive Oil. How much you dilute depends on the particular oil, but starting with a "weak" dilution, and increasing it if needed, is a good rule of thumb. To me, a weak dilution is 1-4 drops per ounce of diluting oil.

There are many ways to apply oils to a pet. You can apply it topically anywhere (except neat in the eyes, into the ear canal, or onto genitals and other sensitive areas). This means a sore knee can have oils applied right to the knee. I have even applied oils to my dog's bald tummy for easy access to a non-furry area! The oils will travel throughout the entire body, and get to where they need to be. Some people even apply oils to their pet's feet. Depending on the pet, this can be an easy or difficult application. In general, I apply to the skin in between the toe pads, and not to the pads themselves. Again, if any irritation is noted (the pet chewing, excessively licking, running around, or any other "frantic" behavior) apply a diluting oil to the site. Then make a note of what dilution you need to use for that particular pet. Individuals can vary – so what is right for one pet may not be right for others.

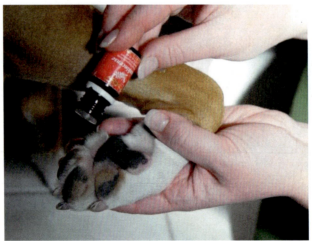

Dripping essential oil onto the foot of a dog.

Tipping the Ears or *Petting the "Cat"* are two of the most popular ways to apply oils. For Tipping the Ears, I generally drip the essential oil into my non-dominant hand and add the diluting oil if necessary. Circle the oils three times clockwise, to energize the oils.

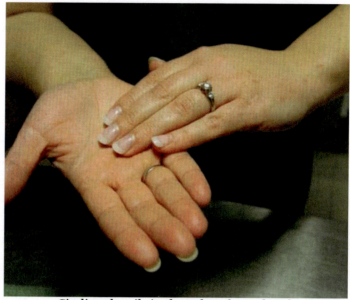
Circling the oils in the palm of your hand.

Then stroke the oils onto the ear flap. I rub the ear between my thumb and forefinger, from base to tip. Careful to not use too much oil – it is okay if your hands actually feel almost dry, but have some scent of the oil on them. This is enough for most animals to have a treatment. Be careful with dogs with very long ears, if they flap their head, they could cause an ear to flip into their eye area – and cause discomfort. Just apply to the base of the ear in long eared pets.

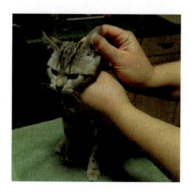
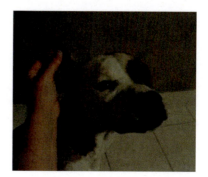

Petting the Cat: Get your oils into your hands as previously described. Then rub your hands together, until there is barely a residue. Then – just pet your Cat (or dog, or even bird, reptile, snake, rat, ferret…). With adding mixing oils to dilute an oil – just be aware that if you use too much – your pet may get greasy. With this method, I have been just fine to apply oils neat to my hands – wait until they are mostly dry – then pet the animal. If you can smell the oil on your hand, you are still giving some therapy to your pet!

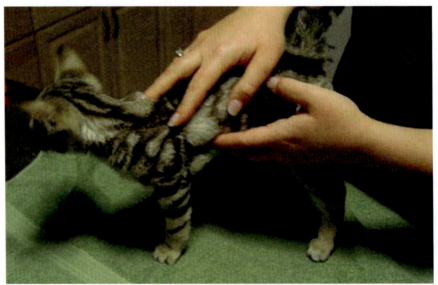

A kitten named "Lavender" having oils applied

Another easy way to apply oils to pets – is with a spritzer bottle. You must use a glass bottle – I use the 4 oz. spray bottle with a trigger sprayer available at www.AbundantHealth4U.com. Add 2-4+ drops of oil to the bottle, and fill the rest of the way with distilled water. Shake before each use, and spritz the area with the very dilute oil. This is also a way to diffuse an oil into the air without a diffuser. Great for safe and healthy bathroom deodorizer too! This is a great way to apply oils to large skin irritations, post surgical areas, feather picking birds, and even some cats.

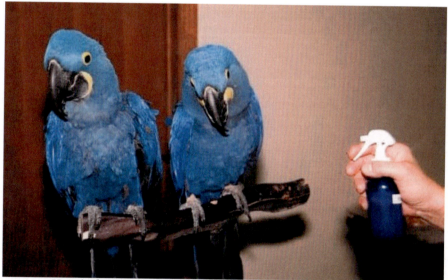

Hyacinth Macaws being spritzed with an Essential Oil solution

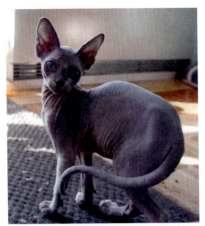
Cats are unique. One might say, they are even from Mars. Their liver enzymes do not metabolize things the same way as a dog or a human. Oils high in eugenol or phenol compounds, can stress their liver. This is even more problematic and even fatal with the use of poor quality, non-medical grade oils. When a pure and medical grade essential oil is collected in its entirety, the trace amounts of chemicals which would normally be missed by the fragrance industry, act as a buffering agent to the rest of the compounds. Basically, if you do not collect the entire oil structure from a plant – you change its chemical make up - thus decreasing the medical benefits, and missing out on some very important properties. It is not always the highest percentage of a chemical that has the medical actions. Sometimes a compound only present at about 1% or less in an oil, is the actual force behind the healing effects.

Oils that are high in phenols and eugenols – are often referred to as "hot" oils. These would be oils that would make you irritated if you touched your face. Common oils to use caution with are: Basil, Cinnamon Bark, Clove, Eucalyptus (all), Lemongrass, Mountain Savory, Oregano, Pepper (Black), Peppermint, Thyme, and Wintergreen.

Of course blended oils containing "hot" oils should also be used with caution. Not that we can't use these oils – we just need to watch closely for reactions (redness, heat, irritation), discomfort, or smell aversions – as well as dilute, dilute, dilute.

The other very important aspect in using oils in animals (especially cats), is to support their system nutritionally. Giving Ningxia Red to animals while they are on essential oils can supply anti-oxidants, and nutrients vital to liver function. Not only will Ningxia Red help *any* health condition by supporting the body – but it is even more critical when we give medications, injections, or even essential oils to sensitive patients. We have noticed that puppies and kittens that get 2-5cc of NingXia Red post vaccination have much less soreness, lethargy or reactions related to vaccination. When I had forgotten to give my own kittens NingXia Red, they limped after a vaccination. Within 1/2 hour of me giving them a dose of Ningxia Red – all limping had stopped.

Essential Oils for Cats

The use of essential oils for cats is the most controversial area in the world of aromatherapy. You will find people who are adamant that essential oils cannot be used safely for cats, and you will find people who are using essential oils daily on their cats. What gives?

The question comes up so many times, over and over again. When I first started into the discovery of essential oils for veterinary use – I immediately went to the internet and searched for animals and essential oils. The information you can find there is scary. "Oils Kill Cats" is a definite theme. However, as I went to more and more classes focusing on the use of oils for humans, I met many people who had not only used essential oils on their cats without killing them, they down right saved their lives with the oils. I had to find out more.

Even my colleagues specializing in holistic medicine warned of the precautions that must be taken when using essential oils in households with felines. But again, here I was, talking with people who had applied the "forbidden oils" directly to their cats – and not only were their cats not dead, but they were also not sick, and were thriving. Many people told stories of how their pets were saved by using a certain essential oil, when a veterinarian had told them it was hopeless.

My mind went crazy! Who was right, and who was wrong. What I quickly found out is that the veterinarians who were so carefully warning other veterinarians and owners not to use essential oils, had in fact, never used them themselves. Now, I try to be open minded, and I admit prior to "finding the oils" I also told my clients that I would "be cautious", and recommended not to use items that I had no knowledge of. That is human nature, to fear the unknown, and avoid it.

I began my journey of researching and learning about these essential oils. What I came to find is that quality does matter. The oils that were linked to killing cats and harming animals were in fact never graded by the veterinarians who condemned them. As all veterinarians know – all medications whether allopathic or alternative – may have side effects. For example, traditional flea and tick medications are very similar to essential oils in regard to quality, effectiveness, and risk. We have seen horrific side effects to the use of over-the-counter, lower cost flea and tick products, and it is not an isolated incident. However, with the use of good quality products (I prefer Frontline Topspot) – I have only seen a handful of "reactions" in 10 years, most amounting to a very minor skin irritation at the site of application. VERY different than the reaction of seizuring and drooling cats, neurologic symptoms, dying kittens, or pets who are frantically trying to rub the product off of themselves.

I look at essential oil brands, much like I look at chemical flea and tick products. You get what you pay for, and you better hope you purchased a good brand! It is not fun to find out that you purchased the "wrong product" after the fact. This is why if I have to use a chemical flea and tick product for a pet – I insist upon it being Frontline. And, if I am going to recommend the use of an essential oil for a pet – it has to be Young Living oils. No exceptions.

So back to the issue of can cats and oils mix? YES, THEY CAN! But, it truly has to be Young Living oils if you are using *any* essential oils in or on *any* pets. This is not a gimmick or a con – this is not a business scheme. This is based on massive amounts of personal and professional research and the veterinary use of essential oils in our practice. I used oils on my own pets (especially cats), before I EVER recommended their use on patients. I monitored laboratory results and health responses to oils extensively.

What is well known in the feline world is that we have to be cautious with the use of essential oils that are high in Phenols and Eugenols. Cats are purely just different. Their liver does not metabolize items the same as a large dog or a human. Dogs can tolerate certain traditional Non-Steroidal Anti-Inflammatories

(NSAIDs). However, given to a cat – you are looking at a likelihood of causing significant damage to organs and even death.

So does this mean that a cat can never be exposed to an oil with Phenols and Eugenols? Oils high in these compounds include "hot" oils such as Oregano, Thyme, Clove, Cinnamon, etc... For a complete listing of oils and their constituents, consult the Essential Oil Desk Reference. No, these oils can be used on cats when needed. If there are other oil choices for treatment that are equally beneficial, I will use those. But when needed and indicated, I know plenty of cats who have had Young Living oils high in phenols and eugenols applied to them quite aggressively, and they did great.

It is important to monitor any animal receiving regular therapies, whether it is with an essential oil or a traditional medication. Blood work before, during, and after application of essential oils and alternative medications, is the only way that we are going to change the mindset of the veterinary world. Gathering important data on the safety and efficacy of alternative treatments falls upon our own shoulders. Drug companies are not interested in natural remedies as they cannot be patented and sold as a monopoly for exorbitant prices.

NingXia Red: While giving oils to cats, it is advisable to give NingXia Red. Some cats love this juice, and others may froth at the mouth. Since I have seen cats do fine during oil use without NingXia Red, I will decide on how important the NingXia Red is to the cat if they are one of those cats that just won't tolerate the NingXia Red. Monitoring blood panels with your veterinarian is a smart decision with any oil use for pets.
- Maintenance Dose: ½ teaspoon once to twice a day.
- During Injury, Illness, or High Oil Usage: 1 Tablespoon or more per day.

The body does best with small, frequent amounts of nutrients. In general, it is far superior to offer NingXia Red 4-6 times a day, than one larger amount once a day. Try offering the NingXia Red straight in a bowl, mixed with canned food, diluted in water, or syringed into the mouth.

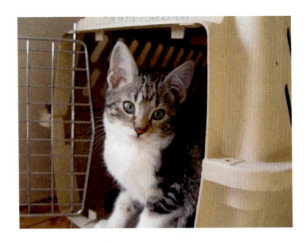

Car Rides: We've all done it. Been in a car with a screaming, meowing cat for what feels like hours. Placing a drop of Lavender on a cotton ball, and placing it inside the carrier has quieted a ride home for many of my clients.

- First Recommendation: Lavender
- Secondary Recommendations: Valerian, Peace & Calming, Sacred Mountain, Valor, Believe

Hairballs: This has to be one of the most common concerns I am asked about. However, although oils can help with this condition – diet is the primary cause for this condition. Changing the diet to a high protein, grain free diet has cured many cats of this chronic condition. Simple allergies to ingredients such as Corn, Soy, Wheat, Dairy, and Egg have caused what we "think" is a hairball. Along with good nutrition, comes less shedding, which is also very helpful in eliminating this annoying situation.

- First Recommendation: Dietary evaluation and changes.
- Secondary Recommendations: DiGize as Litteroma, or applied to feet or abdomen.

Directions: Apply one drop diluted 50:50 with V6 by petting the abdomen or onto the pads of the feet, one to two times a day. Frequency may need to be increased. Further dilution may be indicated if the cat seems uncomfortable from the application of the DiGize Oil.

Litteroma

It remains a fact of life. If you have a cat, you likely have a litter box. Which cat litter to use is often overlooked until your cat is not using the box properly. Besides a complete medical work up to look for health concerns, we also question if the type or brand of kitty litter has recently changed. Certainly we have seen cats stop using a litter box, simply because of a purchase of a new brand of cat litter. Often one that has a strong perfume to it. More concerning is that the use of commercial and fragranced kitty litter has been linked to hyperthyroidism and other health concerns in cats. The chemicals and perfumes within the cat litter, may have detrimental effects over time. I would much rather my cats use a litter box with potential health benefits, instead of concerns. By using essential oils in the kitty litter, I not only have odor controlling properties – but I might also reap the benefits of long term health, prevention of disease, and treatment of medical conditions. Here is one easy way to get your cats some aromatherapy on a regular basis.

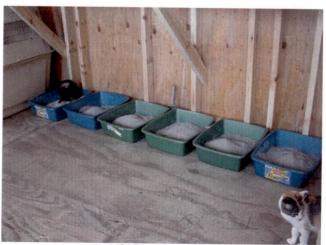

Dr. Shelton's Test Boxes

First, it is very important to make sure that you have clean and new litter boxes. Many people never wash their litter boxes, and never consider that intense urine odors are absorbed by the litter box plastic over time. If your litter box is several years old, chances are you should throw it out and start with a fresh box. I keep several extra litter boxes, so that while one is being washed, a clean one can be used by the cats. Then each box has a chance to air out between uses. Also, covered litter boxes can concentrate odors within the box, leading to a cat that does not want to use a litter box. I compare it to using a biffy or a porta-potty; most of us do not appreciate going into a plastic box, filled with urine and feces. Your cat does not either. Plastic liners can also create a problem for some cats, as when they scratch in the box, their nails can get caught in the liner, causing an aversion for many cats. Box location must also be considered – if you don't like the deep dark basement – why should your cat? And, of course, you must keep your litter box scooped! We certainly bypass an unflushed toilet in the public stalls – why would your cat be any different?

Now that we have addressed some basic litter box guidelines, you can start to play around. Aromatherapy is obviously not just about smelling nice. Classic French aromatherapy is also well known for treating everything from the common cold to arthritis. My theory is that I can have a great smelling litter box, while my cat is enjoying emotional and health benefits of aromatherapy.

Here's how to do it:
1. Place 1 cup of baking soda into a glass jar.

2. Add 1-4+ drops of Young Living Essential Oil to the baking soda.

3. Stir or place the lid onto the jar and shake.

4. Allow to sit overnight to fully disperse the essential oil within the baking soda.

5. Sprinkle into the cat box directly and mix into the UNSCENTED litter (I would generally pick the same litter brand you currently use, just in an unscented version.)

The best way to make sure your cat is happy with your aromatherapy selections, is to give them some choices. When I first started to use this technique, I really wanted to make sure I was not going to offend my cats' delicate sense of smell or pick an oil that they did not like. So I set up a little experiment. I arranged several litter boxes next to each other. In each litter box was a variation, with different types and amounts of essential oils in a different box. I left one box with their regular litter that they were using. You can do your experiment to find out not only which oil your cat will like, but also how many drops of oil to add to the baking soda, and how much baking soda mixture to use per box or litter amount. The combinations are endless, and completely up to you and your cat.

What I found was that my cats actually preferred the boxes with the essential oils in them. This was great proof to me that cats would seek out beneficial aromatherapy if given a choice. Of course, not every cat will be as easy to satisfy as my cats. However, if you give them a choice and they use it – your opportunity to give your cat wonderful benefits of aromatherapy are endless.

Here are some of the oils you could use, and some of the main health benefits associated with them. This is certainly not a complete list of the great attributes of each oil. I encourage everyone to look up their chosen oil(s) in the Essential Oil Desk Reference for full information on each oil or oil blend.

- **Purification:** Mainly picked for odor control in the litter box. However, can also be helpful for respiratory infections, antibacterial properties, insect repellant, and so much more.
- **Copaiba:** Wonderful for arthritis pain and inflamed bladders.
- **Myrrh, EndoFlex or Frankincense:** Beneficial for hyperthyroid conditions.
- **Ocotea:** Diabetes.
- **Frankincense:** Anti-Cancer properties, age related changes, senility...
- **DiGize:** Hairballs, diarrhea, or parasite concerns.

The list is really never-ending. Rotating through several oil selections is likely to be the best way to ensure that your cat is receiving long term and broad based benefits. Give it a try, and see what your cat thinks!

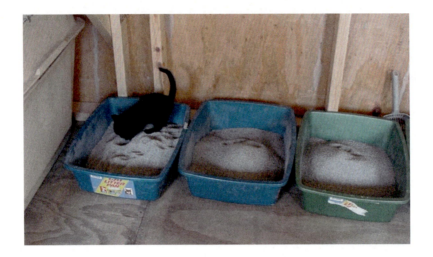

Respiratory Conditions

Cats are famous for Upper Respiratory Infections or URI's. Almost everyone has had a cat with the sneezes or some nasal discharge. Sometimes this can become a chronic condition. URI's can be caused by bacteria or by viruses in cats. By using essential oils that address both anti-bacterial properties and anti-viral properties, we benefit the cats in many ways.

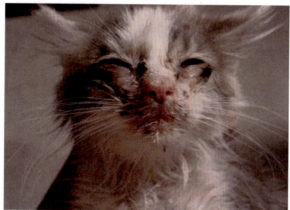

"Sweet Pea" – a rescued kitten with a severe Upper Respiratory Infection

Diffusion is my favorite method for administering essential oils in this condition. Placing the kitten into a carrier, and using a water-based ultrasonic style diffuser. Sometimes I will place a towel or plastic wrap over the carrier and diffuser; creating a "tent" which will trap the beneficial vapors within the carrier.

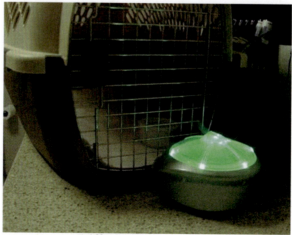

Diffusing into a carrier.

- First Recommendations: Purification with Eucalyptus Blue.
- Secondary Recommendations: Thieves, RC, Pine – also diffused with Eucalyptus Blue.

In an average ultrasonic diffuser, place 4-8 drops of Purification and 2 drops of Eucalyptus Blue. Starting with a lower concentration and gradually increasing the intensity as needed is a great way to start.

- Nutritional Notes: Often cats with frustrating chronic upper respiratory infections are found to have nutritional deficiencies. Whole food supplements have been incredibly important in allowing the body to achieve full healing. Young Living supplements such as Multigreens, NingXia Red, and True Source can be incredibly beneficial, however they are vegetarian based. Many cats will only completely heal and resolve a chronic issue with supplements formulated directly for the carnivorous nature of cats. Recommended supplements are Feline Whole Body Support and Feline Immune Support. Please see the chapter on Whole Food Supplements for more information on this subject as well as ordering advice.

Multigreens: Generally open a capsule and mix into canned food. Start with a small amount (just a sprinkling) for picky cats, and gradually increase the amount given. Generally, work up to using 1 capsule per day. However, in severe cases two or more capsules may be used. The Melissa oil contained within this supplement is the highest anti-viral oil. This supplement is indicated for any cat dealing with a viral infection of any nature (and especially in cats with chronic Herpes Virus).

NingXia Red: Follow the guidelines on page 38 for dosing information.

True Source: This supplement comes in a little pouch containing three different colored whole food supplements. Open one capsule and mix the some of the contents into canned food. Mixing supplements into Chicken Baby Food is also widely accepted and enjoyed by cats. Rotate through which "colored" capsule is given, and generally work up to giving one full capsule per day. Start with a small sprinkling, and gradually increase the amount fed until you are giving up to ½ of a capsule at a feeding. This supplement is helpful in those kitties who crave eating grass.

Abscesses

Cat bites are often the cause of an abscess in a cat. They become infected, painful, and can cause high fever and illness in under an hour. ALWAYS SEEK THE ATTENTION OF A VETERINARIAN AS SOON AS POSSIBLE. In severe situations, veterinary care is of the utmost importance – and use of oral antibiotics should not be foregone if needed. I have seen cats spike a fever to over 105 degrees Fahrenheit from a "simple" cat fight wound. Drainage of the pus is important.

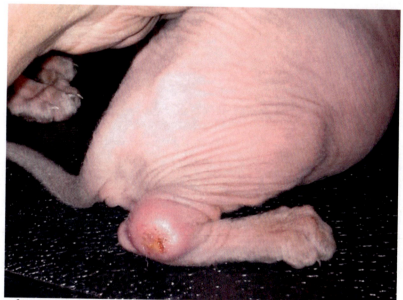

An abscess on the right rear leg of a Sphynx kitten – appropriately named "Rose"

The particular kitten in the picture above was placed on oral antibiotics. An abscess involving a joint area is nothing to mess around with. However, Lavender and Purification Oils were also applied neat to the area several times a day. We believe we saw a larger response to the oils, than to the actual oral antibiotics. It is wonderful to know that we can, and should, support our animals with allopathic and alternative healing methods when needed. I am certain that the inflammation and wound healed quicker, and she was more able to deal with any possible side effects of the oral antibiotics due to our holistic treatment of this wound.

- <u>First Recommendation</u>: Purification, Lauris Nobilis
- <u>Secondary Recommendations</u>: Melrose, Egyptian Gold, Spikenard, Animal Scents Ointment, Animal Scents Shampoo, Thieves Household Cleaner, Kitty Raindrop Technique

<u>Directions</u>: Apply the chosen oil neat (or undiluted) directly onto the abscess "head", if the abscess has not broken open yet. The "head" is the location where it looks like the abscess is about ready to pop on its own. You can see that "Rose's" abscess has not broken open, and still contains a "head". If the cat seems uncomfortable with the application, or excessive irritation of the skin seems to follow the application – dilute the oil with V6 prior to application. This is more important with Egyptian Gold, which contains Cinnamon Bark – a "hot" oil. When diluting – I try to dilute as little as possible to the point where irritation does not occur. Or, I may try an application where I apply the oil neat to the abscess at first, but then immediately follow the essential oil with V6, to dilute it immediately after "neat" penetration.

Apply the oil neat to the abscess, generally twice a day until the wound breaks open. You can also apply a hot pack, saturated with the solution described below to the abscess area. This can help a scab or debris to be removed from the abscess head.

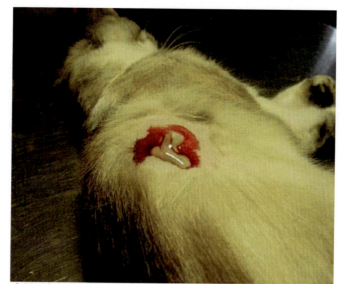
A cat bite abscess, lanced and draining at the Veterinary Hospital.

If the abscess has already started to drain, or it is "empty" – add 2-4 drops of the chosen essential oil to a teaspoon of Animal Scents Shampoo, Thieves Household Cleaner, Young Living Bath Gel Base, or (in a pinch) even one of the Young Living Shampoos. Dilute your essential oil/soap base in 2-4 cups of warm water or saline (DO NOT WARM YOUR WATER OR SALINE IN A MICROWAVE). You want the solution to disinfect the wound, however not be so soapy as to irritate or leave a residue. To test the solution, "wash" your hands with the solution, but do not rinse or dry them. If you feel sticky or like you would like to wash it off your hands – then dilute the solution further.

Use a syringe to irrigate and flush the open and draining abscess. Repeat the irrigation several times until the pus is gone and the wound is relatively clean. If there is excessive residue – rinse with plain warm water or saline. However, the goal is to leave a small amount of the disinfecting solution within the walls of the abscess.

Irrigation may be painful to your cat, especially if you force the issue. Once an abscess has opened on its own, irrigation is not as likely to be uncomfortable. The Thieves Household Cleaner based solution is most likely to reduce discomfort, as it contains topically anesthetic essential oils. Repeat irrigation once or twice a day, until no further pus is draining from the site. ALWAYS

SEEK THE ATTENTION OF A VETERINARIAN FOR ANY CAT BITE ABSCESS AS SOON AS POSSIBLE.

Once you no longer need to irrigate the wound, you can hot pack the area with the same irrigation solution. This will help you to keep the area clean and aid in healing. Use a washcloth with as hot of solution as you can comfortably stand on your bare skin for at least 20 seconds or longer. Never use a microwave to heat this solution. Warm your water on the stove, or I use a coffee maker to keep hot water available to me at all times (no coffee, just run water through). Add your essential oil/soap to the pleasantly hot water. Wring out the excess solution from your washcloth, but leave it somewhat moist. Hold the hot washcloth over the abscess until the heat is gone. Use the washcloth to gently cleanse the area, removing any old scabby debris, dried pus, or dead skin. Hot pack the area 2-3 times a day or as needed to keep the area clean.

Essential Oils orally for cats: While this certainly can be done, many cats remain quite difficult to administer oral oils to. Lauris Nobilis would be my first choice of an oil to use orally for a cat. Oils dripped directly into the mouth, is the ideal method to give oils orally. Secondarily, placing the oil within a capsule and "pilling" the cat is another option, however slightly less effective due to the digestive process. One drop, 2-4 times a day would be a starting point for most cats. If vomiting, lethargy, or diarrhea is noted – stopping or reducing the dosage is advisable. I recommend that any cat getting treated "aggressively" with essential oils, be monitored with a blood panel and CBC in cooperation with a veterinarian, as well as to make sure that the cat is fully hydrated prior to the treatment. Giving an already dehydrated and sick cat large amounts of essential oils, can detoxify their body more than they can handle comfortably. NingXia Red should be given as well, for additional support. For me, I will still choose to treat cat abscesses with traditional antibiotics as well as essential oils, however, there is an occasional cat who cannot tolerate oral antibiotics – and it is wonderful that there are other choices that can be made.

Kitty Raindrop Technique (KRDT)

Directions for Kitty Raindrop Technique (adapted from Leigh Foster):

1. In a one ounce (30mL) glass bottle (empty essential oil bottles are available at www.AbundantHealth4u.com) – mix 4 drops of each of the following oils:
    Oregano
    Thyme
    Basil
    Cypress
    Wintergreen
    Marjoram
    Peppermint

2. Optional: 2-4 drops of DiGize oil can also be added to this mixture – it is not part of the Raindrop Technique per se, but cats often benefit from this oil. DiGize is often used for gastro-intestinal upset, parasites, and hairballs.

3. Fill the bottle the rest of the way with Young Living V6 diluting oil. I prefer V6 over Olive Oil as it is thinner and seems to be more "user friendly" on a furry being. Mix this solution well.

4. Optional: In another bottle, create a diluted version of Valor. Leigh recommends diluting it 50:50 with V6. I usually use Valor neat (or undiluted).

5. Optional: Tip the ears of the cat with Lavender angustifolia oil, and/or apply it to yourself. This will help calm the cat for the Raindrop application (as well as you).

You are now ready to apply the Kitty Raindrop Technique:

1. Once the kitty is calm, tip the ears of the cat with the diluted Valor mixture (optional step). Then place a few drops of Valor (diluted or neat) into each hand, rub together, and then balance the cat or kitten's energy by placing your hands on the base of the neck and at the base of the tail. Take deep breaths; relaxing, calming, and meditating. ☺ This is good for you and the cat!

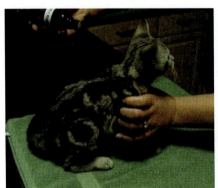 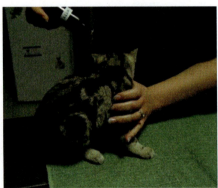

"Lavender" the kitten getting her drops.

2. When you and the cat are ready, drip about 6 drops of the KRDT oil mixture along the spine, starting at the tail and going to the base of the head. Then massage in the oil (with classic feathering strokes), working from the base of the tail to the base of the head. While you are massaging, you can start to part the fur down the spine, although it is not necessary. Depending on the cat, I have had to just "pet" and massage the oils into the back from head to tail. It purely depends on the cat - if they appreciate their hair being rubbed the "wrong way" or not. I will apply the oils "backwards" or "forwards" to adjust to the individual cat.

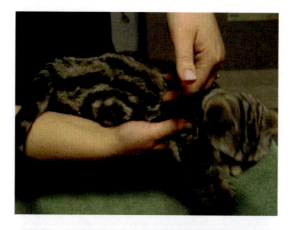

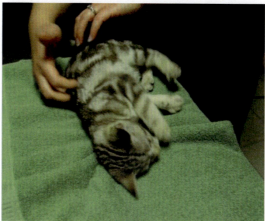

"Lavender" is a bit of a moving target!

3. When indicated, repeat applying about 6 drops of the KRDT oil mixture down the parted area of the spine. Continue to massage gently. Usually, the cat will start to relax and "melt" into the massage. Continue to apply the oils 6 drops at a time along the spine and massaging until the animal lets you know (or you feel that) it is enough. Often I find that 1-3 applications is about right (so about 6-18 drops of the KRDT solution total). Although there are certain cats that beg for the oil to be applied over and over again, I usually limit their enjoyment until I see their response to the KRDT.

4. If possible, I will VitaFlex up the kitty's back (three times if permitted). Again, this depends on what the cat feels like allowing. But it is a wonderful addition if you can include it.

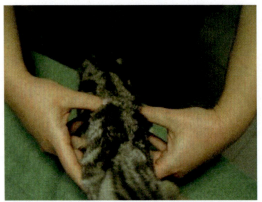

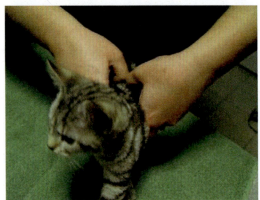

VitaFlex with the thumbs, up the back. From tail to head.

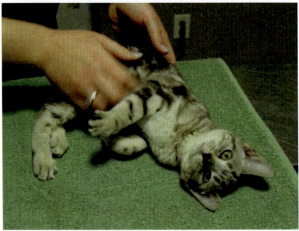

All done! One happy kitten!

I have used a Kitty Raindrop Technique daily, and now even twice a day in cats that have a severe medical concern. Leigh Foster has used this application to help clear Feline Leukemia and FIV from her rescued cats. When using the Raindrop for this purpose, she applies it every day until the virus is cleared, retesting every 1-2 months with her veterinarian. She also uses the KRDT weekly in feral cats to help calm and domesticate them. In her healthy cats, she applies a KRDT once a month just for maintenance and because they love it.

Who is a Raindrop For?
Who *Isn't* a Raindrop For!

When you consider all of the oils that are a part of a Raindrop Technique – it is hard to imagine an animal (or person for that matter) that wouldn't benefit from a Raindrop Technique! Just look at the properties listed for each oil – direct from the Essential Oils Desk Reference:

- <u>Oregano</u>: anti-aging, powerful anti-viral, antibacterial, antifungal, antiparasitic, anti-inflammatory, immune stimulant
- <u>Thyme</u>: anti-aging, highly anti-microbial, antifungal, antiviral, antiparasitic.
- <u>Basil</u>: Anti-spasmodic, antiviral, antibacterial, anti-inflammatory, muscle relaxant, anti-histamine
- <u>Cypress</u>: Improves circulation, strengthens capillaries, anti-infectious, anti-spasmodic, discourages fluid retention
- <u>Wintergreen</u>: Anticoagulant, antispasmodic, highly anti-inflammatory, vasodilator, analgesic/anesthetic, reduces blood pressure, all types of pain, musculoskeletal problems.
- <u>Marjoram</u>: Muscle soothing, relieve body and joint discomfort, soothe digestive tract, antibacterial, antifungal, vasodilator, lowers blood pressure, promotes intestinal peristalsis, expectorant, mucolytic
- <u>Peppermint</u>: Driving Oil. Anti-inflammatory, antitumoral, antiparasitic (worms), antibacterial, antiviral, antifungal, gall bladder/digestive stimulant, pain-relieving.

Ear Mites

Any discharge within a cat's ear is not normal. If your cat has ear debris, you should have an ear smear completed by your veterinarian to see if the infection is mites, bacteria, or yeast. Treatments will vary depending on the cause. Killing ear mites with natural remedies takes more dedication and commitment than using traditional veterinary chemicals. If ear mites have not cleared up within 1 month, or your cat is having difficulties being treated, or cannot tolerate the oil application – treating ear mites allopathically is recommended. My first traditional recommendation is Revolution.

- <u>First Recommendation</u>: Purification
- <u>Second Recommendation</u>: Peppermint

Directions and Comments:
- Start by cleaning the ears. Apply Organic Coconut Oil, coating the inside of the ear and its "nooks and crannies". This will help dissolve and break up the black waxy areas, allowing them to be scooped out more effectively and gently. Swab out as much debris as possible, as gently as possible, with a cotton swab. It is not uncommon for ears that are infected with ear mites, to bleed slightly as you clean due to all of the existing irritation. Many cats scratch frantically during the cleaning – do not confuse the irritation of the ear mite condition itself, with irritation by the essential oil. However, when in doubt – assume that the essential oil may be causing additional temporary discomfort, and dilute the oil or apply additional carrier oil after application.

- Apply 1-2 drops of the essential oil to a cotton swab, and swab the inside of the ear. DO NOT DRIP OILS DIRECTLY INTO THE EAR CANAL. Repeat once or twice a day for 10-14 days, or until the ear mites are gone. Check the ears for irritation after application – slight discomfort and dislike of the oil in the ear is expected for a short time. However if the ears are hot or red, or the cat shows agitation for longer than 15-30 seconds – apply a carrier such as V6 to the ears. Most of the time, if the ear was cleaned with Coconut oil prior to the application of the essential oil, there will already be a "protective" coating of carrier oil within the ear, and irritation is less likely. Dilute the essential oil with V6 prior to future applications if any irritation is noted. I generally start with diluting 1 drop of essential oil with 1 drop of V6. Dilute further if irritation is still noted with that dilution.

- Recheck an ear smear with your veterinarian to ensure that the mites have been eliminated.

Feline Leukemia:

Feline leukemia is a devastating virus for cats, often leading to death. Unfortunately, many cats are never given the chance for recovery. Once a positive test result is found, many veterinarians are quick to recommend euthanasia. Thankfully, there are some holistic vets who have seen more and more cats and kittens recover from this virus, and regain a negative test result. If you happen to have a cat or kitten that tests positive for Feline Leukemia, I encourage you to keep them isolated from other cats, do not allow them to go outdoors, and to start a nutritional and holistic care regimen that can allow the body to clear the virus. Retest with your veterinarian every 1-3 months, but allow a full 6 months for results to fully change. It may not be every cat that can convert to a negative status – but in our animal hospital, we have certainly seen the vast majority of kittens dealing with this virus, have converted to negative test results.

- First Recommendations: Kitty Raindrop Technique, Melissa, Frankincense, Hyssop, Multigreens, NingXia Red
- Secondary Recommendations: Eucalyptus Blue, Copaiba as a magnifier oil

Administer the KRDT daily. Additionally add 4 drops of each of the first recommendation oils and 4 drops of Copaiba to the KRDT Solution. For some cats, an increase of some oils may be indicated. Adjust oil concentrations more or less depending on the cat's response.

Diffuse first and secondary recommendation oils as much as possible. I like to mix a couple together, and sometimes with other oils not listed. For example – I may diffuse Purification and add a couple of drops of Frankincense and Copaiba to that diffusion. Or, I may diffuse Thieves with some Eucalyptus Blue and Copaiba. I try to diffuse as much as possible in the area that the cat is in. I generally use an ultrasonic diffuser with cats; however you could use an air diffuser. With air diffusers – make sure that the concentration of the oil vapors do not become too concentrated in a closed location with the cat. Certainly, contact with oils being injected directly into the air – could cause some eye or mucus membrane discomfort.

Give NingXia Red in fairly high doses. You may need to gradually increase the amount for some cats, or hide within food. Split 1-2 Tablespoons per day, into several doses. An amino acid called "DMG" has been shown to be helpful in clearing feline leukemia virus from cats. NingXia Red is a wonderful source of amino acids.

Give 1-2 capsules of Multigreens per day. Open the capsule and mix with canned or fresh foods. Gradually increase the amount given, to make sure the cat can tolerate it. Multigreens contain Melissa oil, so are an affordable way to include this oil into your regimen.

Vitamin E: Human Vitamin E capsules can be purchased and popped with a pin. 1-2 drops twice a day on food or directly into the mouth is an incredibly immune supportive regimen.

Whole Food Supplements: Standard Process Feline Whole Body Support and Feline Immune Support are both well indicated.

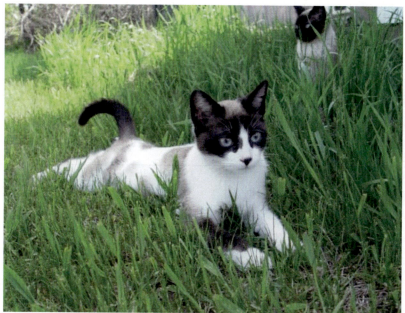

Outdoor cats are much more likely to contract Feline Leukemia. Infections mainly occur in cats under one year of age. Natural resistance is high in cats older than one year.

DOGS:

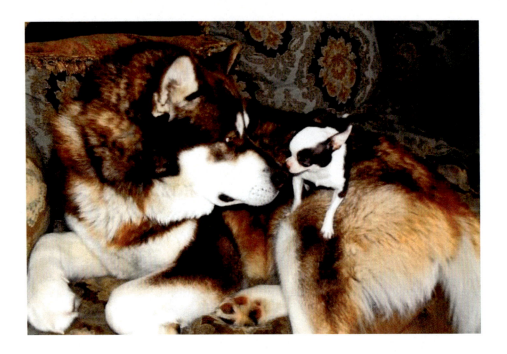

Dogs come in all shapes and sizes. To make dosing as easy as possible, please refer to these approximate sizes of dogs.

Small Dog: 1-20 Pounds (0-9 kg)
Medium: 20-50 Pounds (9-22 kg)
Large: 50-100 Pounds (23-45 kg)
X-Large: 100+ Pounds (45+ kg)

Arthritis

Arthritis is a common issue these days, but what is arthritis? Arthritis is inflammation in and around the joints. Any joint can be affected – even jaws, vertebrae, tails, and toes. It is not always just a hip, elbow, or shoulder joint that is affected, although these are the most common. Arthritis is a vicious cycle, and once the body becomes inflamed, the body sends out messages to "stabilize" the condition. This is generally attempted by the laying down of more bone and unfortunately more inflammation. Sometimes we get a condition called an osteophyte – which is a boney growth off of the bone itself.

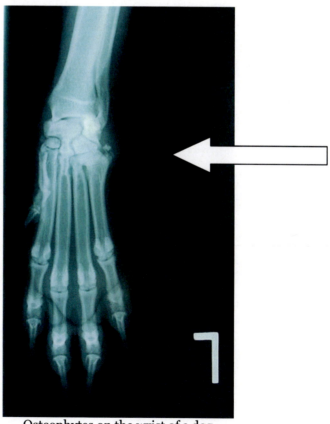

Osteophytes on the wrist of a dog

More inflammation means more arthritis. More arthritis means more inflammation. It becomes a horrible snowball effect. Often times when pets become painful, we turn towards chronic administration of Non-Steroidal Anti-inflammatories (NSAIDs). Not only can NSAIDs be expensive, but they can be detrimental to your pet's health. Blood tests are recommended before, during, and after the use of many of these popular traditional drugs – and for good reason. Even dog-specific "safe" NSAIDs can be incredibly hard on the liver.

Prevention of arthritis is largely ignored in the veterinary and animal community. In our veterinary clinic, when we start an older dog with arthritis on essential oils and supplements for arthritis they have near miraculous results, and start moving easier and feeling better. My theory has always been that if we can give an older animal comfort once they are already arthritic…what could we do if we started these supplements much earlier? My own dogs are given joint supplements from the moment they join our family. With one of our dogs, he started taking supplements when he was 7 weeks old. Currently at 7 years old, he has experienced injuries that should have greatly increased his chances of arthritis. From being run over by a large SUV to fracturing a leg…we saw him heal faster and easier than any dog I have ever seen. He is amazingly active, and although I can't prove it, I believe that holistic care, oils, and supplements have contributed to his amazing health and well being.

What will your pet or animal show you when they have arthritis? Unfortunately, the symptoms are wide and varied. We see anything from less activity, to limping, to intermittent and occasional limping. We have even seen poor and finicky eating, shaking, fevers, reluctance to put their head down (which can relate to the poor appetite as well when the food bowl is placed low). The hard part for me – is that many owners just expect that their pet is getting older, and that laying around is normal for them. But then when we start them on a protocol to help with inflammation, arthritis, and joint health – they start dragging their owner on a walk again.

If you have an older dog, who you think might "just be getting old" – starting him on an arthritis regimen for 3-6 weeks, can help you evaluate if your dog has unrecognized discomfort. When addressing the arthritis with nutrition, it is important to allow enough time for nutrients to be absorbed and to change the situation. Essential oils alone can relieve inflammation more quickly, but it is important to allow enough time to fully evaluate if your dog is feeling better.

So let's go over the basics of what I see are important with arthritis. All of these are part of how I treat arthritis – but it is my belief that if pets were to get these things in their lives on a daily basis, we will have arthritis prevention instead of treatment. I would much rather consult with people on well care, than on sick care!

Diet is obviously an important aspect of our pet's health. Junky diets are obviously going to be causing health issues and limit the amount of healing that your pet can achieve. All food sources are deficient in vitamins, minerals and enzymes these days. Our soil is depleted, and even on a raw diet that should contain more enzymes and unharmed nutrients – we will never be perfect in this day and age. Our foods just can't have the same nutritional value that they did years ago, and all of our food supplies are certainly exposed to pollution and toxins that we just didn't have 50 years ago. And, certainly not in the quantities that we have today. I believe that all diets should be supplemented with a digestive enzyme. Protein digestion is one of the main areas shown to correlate with arthritis inflammation. Adding an enzyme like Polyzyme that is directed toward protein digestion is very important for our carnivorous pets who are fed processed foods. Allerzyme and Mightyzymes also have great general spectrums for digestion as well. All of the Young Living enzymes are wonderful.

Hydration is important to everyone. But often times our senior pets are also dehydrated. They need more moisture to feel better, have healthier muscles, and more lubricated joint fluids. Adding water to their dry kibble, or extra water to moist food – should be a main stay. Raw diets are naturally high in moisture content, and do a great job of keeping pets hydrated.

Omega Fatty Acids are next on the list. Omega Blue from Young Living is a great supplement. Not only do they contain high quality fatty acids, but they also contain essential oils that prevent rancidity and have other health benefits as well. The EPA component within Omega 3 fatty acids also acts to shut off arthritis feed back. So as the arthritis inflammation is telling the body to react more, and make the condition worse – EPA shuts that down. Omega's also have anti-inflammatory actions on their own.

Sulfurzyme is another very important recommendation. Sulfurzyme contains MSM and NingXia Wolfberries. MSM is a natural source of sulfur, which is an important part of every cell in our body. It is not the same as "Sulfa" – like the antibiotics. Sulfur is totally different. Sulfur is necessary for our bodies to function, and we are likely very deficient in it. MSM is also a natural anti-inflammatory. However, it has been shown that it needs Vitamin C in order for it to be absorbed by the body. This is why I have so many clients that have tried a joint supplement and have seen no benefits. Usually it is a product that is not bio-available at all. So this means that you now just have expensive poop, that didn't really help your dog's arthritis. Sulfurzyme comes in capsules and powder – and is very well accepted by pets. The NingXia Wolfberry alone has many health benefits, but also provides the Vitamin C necessary for the MSM to work to full effect. I continually see pets respond quickly and wonderfully to the Sulfurzyme. It is not just for arthritis...Sulfurzyme can be helpful for surgical healing, scar tissue, skin issues, and so much more!

One of the other problems with processed dog foods is that it is very deficient in cartilaginous materials. It sounds really nice that our pet foods are made with human quality meats – but this means that the pets are mainly getting muscle tissue. Gone are the meaty chewy parts that animals treasure, the sinewy tendons and ligaments, the grizzly cartilage. If you ask your dog, they would love to chew on a raw meaty bone; with cartilage and muscle, sinew, and bone marrow. The thing we need to remember is that the nutrients that are most necessary for bone, are found in bone. The nutrients that are needed for cartilage, are found in cartilage. This is true for all of the organs as well. Animals used to eat organ meats, and knuckle bones – and they don't get it anymore. So if we want healthy cartilage, we are going to need to supplement for it. BLM Capsules from Young Living contain glucosamine and chondroitin, as well as wintergreen and other essential oils beneficial for bones, joints and ligaments. One important thing to note – is that the BLM Powder contains xylitol. Xylitol has been linked to hypoglycemia and liver concerns in certain dogs who have consumed it. So I recommend using the BLM Capsules to avoid any cause for concern. In recommended dosages, you are unlikely to have an issue, but since there is an alternative – I would recommend using the safer avenue. I generally just open the capsule and sprinkle it into food. If the dog is large enough you may just give the capsule whole.

When an animal actually needs an anti-inflammatory – then Copaiba is my oil. I have seen so many amazing things. It is the highest anti-inflammatory oil, and may surpass cortisone, aspirin, ibuprofen, or acetaminophen in action. These items can be down right fatal to an animal; however Copaiba has very little if any side effects at all. Even one small baby aspirin is enough to cause a stomach ulcer in a dog's stomach. Copaiba just happens to be gastro-protective as well! How great is that? It can decrease inflammation, as well as protect the gut from ulcers! In veterinary school, I was taught of a study in dogs where aspirin was given to dogs and then they were examined with an endoscope to view the inside of the stomach. Over 90% of all dogs, even if they had only received small doses for a few days – had gastric ulcers – or ulcers inside their stomach! I see so many older farm dogs on aspirin – and it is slowly killing them. And then when the ulcer becomes severe, they end up very ill, and hospitalized, sometimes to the tune of hundreds to thousands of dollars. So a small investment in a bottle of copaiba oil is a no brainer. There is 285 drops in general, in a 15 mL bottle – even in a large dog – I usually use 1-2 drops twice a day or less. This would provide 2-4 months of use! This is far more affordable than prescription NSAIDs that we use in pets. What I enjoy most about this oil, is that it can be used with other veterinary drugs. So even if a dog is on other medications, even NSAIDs or steroids, I can safely transition them to using Copaiba, without worrying about drug interactions.

- <u>First Recommendations</u>: Copaiba, Sulfurzyme, BLM Capsules, Omega Blue, Polyzyme, Frankincense
- <u>Secondary Recommendations</u>: PanAway, Regenolone Cream, Ortho Ease, Ortho Sport, Lemongrass, Wintergreen, Idaho Balsam Fir, NingXia Red, Palo Santo, RC (for osteophytes)

General Recommendations: Copaiba with Arthritis –
- Small dogs: mix 1 part Copaiba with 3 parts V6 – for example – 1 drop of copaiba with 3 drops of V6 diluting oil. Then give 1-2 drops of this dilution, twice a day. This oil can be fed in food, given directly orally, or applied topically in almost any location. It could also be mixed with a small amount of NingXia Red and administered in the juice.
- Medium Dogs: mix 1 part Copaiba with 1 part V6. Give 1-2 drops of this dilution, twice a day.
- Large Dogs: give 1 drop of Copaiba without dilution, twice a day.

After a period of 1-2 months, I often find that the amount of Copaiba needed to maintain comfort is lessened. Many of my clients have diluted their Copaiba oil in half, and have continued to see the awesome benefits from the "half dosage".

Sulfurzyme – Thankfully, it is almost impossible to give too much of this supplement. If you do, you will see soft stools. Start with a lower dose, and slowly work up. One Capsule = ¼ teaspoon of powder. The doses below are the general maximum dosages, your dog may feel benefits with less.

- Small dog – 1 – 1 ½ tsp. once to twice a day
- Medium dog – 1 heaping tsp.
- Large dog – 1 heaping Tbsp.

Incontinence (Urinary)

Urinary incontinence is most commonly seen in older, spayed female dogs. These dogs typically leak urine, especially while sleeping.

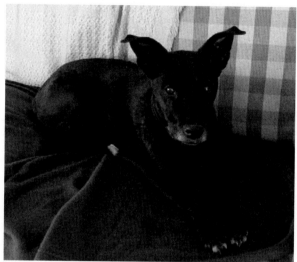

"Q" our 15 ½ year old dog, who taught us so much about Copaiba, Arthritis, and Incontinence!

<u>First Recommendation</u>: Copaiba
<u>Secondary Recommendations</u>: NingXia Red, Omega Blue, Sulfurzyme

Directions:
- Small and Medium Dogs – dilute Copaiba with an equal part of V6 or Olive Oil. Give 1 drop twice a day by mouth, in food, or on skin.
- Large Dogs – 1 drop twice a day, generally neat by mouth, in food, or on skin.

It may take up to one month to see full results. When dogs are on medications for this problem, I use the essential oils and supplements for approximately one month, and work with a veterinarian to gradually reduce the medications being given for incontinence, while continuing the essential oil.

Copaiba is generally a very mild oil. It has very little taste and has been easily accepted in dog's food. Only very rarely, have I ever seen a skin sensitivity to Copaiba oil.

Ear Infections

It is not normal for there to be any colored wax or debris in a dog's ear. If there is a dark substance in the ear at all, this is a sign of an infection. Most dogs will have yeast (fungal) or bacterial infections in the ear, with yeast being the most common. Bacterial infections tend to be more painful, and have a more "slimy" discharge. Dogs with ear infections often shake their heads and may cry out when their ears are touched. Ear mites do occur in dogs, but it is less common than in cats.

It is very important to have your veterinarian help you diagnose what type of ear infection your dog has. You want to make sure that your veterinarian performs an "Ear Smear" and examines the debris under a microscope to look for bacteria, yeast, or mites. However, ear infections often "pop up" on weekends or when you can't get into the veterinarian in a timely manner. Gently cleaning the ears and offering some relief to the pet can be a great thing until you can get into the veterinarian.

Ear Cleaning…The Natural Way

An all natural ear cleaner can be made from a very diluted solution of Thieves Household Cleaner or Animal Scents Shampoo. Although we should never put neat, or undiluted, essential oils directly into the ear (dripping oils down into the ear canal) – they can be used in cleaning solutions, ointments, and other ear treatments. Even the mainstream veterinary world is using essential oils in many ear care products.

- To start add 1 teaspoon of Thieves Household Cleaner or Animal Scents Shampoo to 4 cups of warm water. The solution can be made stronger or weaker if needed. If the ear gets sudsy and foamy, dilute your solution more.
- Optional: Add 2-4 Tablespoons of Organic Apple Cider Vinegar to the wash solution. Vinegar is naturally antifungal and can help fight yeast.
- Optional: Add 2-4 drops of essential oil(s) to the teaspoon of Thieves Household Cleaner or Animal Scents Shampoo and combine well. Then mix this solution into the warm water. The cleaner and shampoo act as a carrier and helps to disperse the essential oil within the ear cleaner.

Coconut Oil is a gentle and effective ear cleaner that has therapeutic benefits. Waxy debris dissolves easily within the oil and helps you to gently clean it away. It also has natural antifungal and antibacterial properties, which will help with an ear infection.

I prefer to use Nutiva Raw Organic Coconut Oil, which is available at www.Nutiva.com. Wholesale ordering is also available for businesses.

Coconut Oil is solid at room temperature, then melts at body temperature.
Small amounts of Essential Oils can be mixed into the softened, liquid Coconut Oil to allow for extra benefits during cleansing. You can then allow the Coconut Oil to "set up" again. Then, take a dollop of the "oiled" coconut oil, and use this to clean or treat the ears.

Oil Suggestions: Purification, Melrose, Thieves, Lavendula angustifolia (Lavender), Copaiba, Melaleuca alternifolia (Tea Tree).

Ear Spray Recipe

This ear spray was developed by Sara Kenney, and is so wonderful that your veterinarian may not have much to look at after a few days of use! Sara's website is www.SaraLivingWell.com.

In a 1 ounce (30 mL) glass spray or dropper bottle add:

- 1 ½ teaspoons of Thieves Essential Oil Blend Spray
- 1 Tablespoon of Young Living V6 Diluting Oil
- 3 Drops of Lemongrass Essential Oil
- 4 Drops of Copaiba Essential Oil
- 5 Drops of Purification Essential Oil Blend

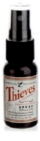

Add distilled water to fill the bottle. Spray into ears as needed, generally once or twice a day with severe irritation. The V6 Diluting Oil is much thinner and sprays out of a spray bottle easier. If using a dropper bottle, gently apply the solution to the outer part of the ear, and do not drip large amounts directly down into the ear canal.

This spray has properties that help fight bacteria and yeast without the risks of bacterial resistance to antibiotics. Since each plant crop is slightly different, each essential oil will be slightly different upon distillation. Bacteria cannot adapt to these constant variations, and therefore do not develop resistance to most plant molecules.

First Recommendations:
- Ear Spray Recipe
- Consult a holistic veterinarian to find the underlying cause of the ear infection.

Secondary Recommendations:
- Place 1-2 drops of Melrose or Purification onto a cotton ball. Place inside the ear. Change twice a day for 3-5 days.
- Inner Defense – for severe infections.
  - Small Dog: start with one capsule per day.
  - Medium Dog: 1-2 capsules per day.
  - Large Dog: 1-3 capsules per day.

Cruciate Injuries (Knee Injury)

The Cruciate Ligaments are located inside the canine stifle (knee). The Cranial Cruciate Ligament is the same ligament referred to as the Anterior Cruciate Ligament (ACL) in humans – and is the most commonly injured ligament in the knee. It helps to stabilize the knee as it moves. Canines and humans alike can injure this ligament, and it causes pain and instability inside the knee. Sometimes the cartilage inside the knee is also damaged when this ligament becomes damaged. Often times we hear from a client that their dog was just fine one minute, went outside to go potty, and came in only walking on three of their legs.

Many times these dogs do not act painful, as they still happily run around on the other three legs. This is confusing to most owners, as the condition does not "seem" painful – but I assure you that it is, and that is why these dogs will not use the affected leg(s).

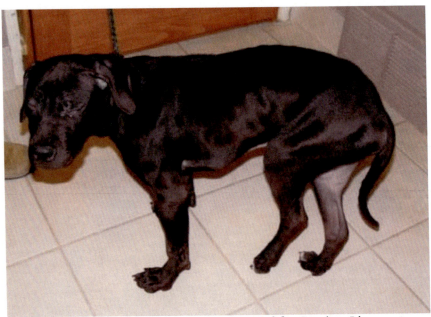

"Buddy" a rescued dog with a partial tear of the Cruciate Ligaments
This leg position is typical of a knee injury.

A veterinarian will feel for signs of laxity within the joint, referred to as a "drawer sign", to diagnose this problem. Radiographs can be helpful however do not truly diagnose the injury. They only support the findings of the injury. A dog can have a partial tear or a complete tear of the Cruciate Ligament. A partial tear will often not have an obvious "drawer sign", and is much more amenable to medical treatment. Often times, surgery is recommended for a complete tear – although I have seen dogs diagnosed with complete tears that did still heal with conservative treatment. Since we cannot truly evaluate the level of the tear without surgery or endoscopic examination inside of the knee – it is hard to know for sure to what level there are still ligament fibers intact within the knee.

If I cannot feel a significant amount of "drawer sign" within a knee – I choose a conservative approach for 1-3 months and see what response is made.

First Recommendations:
- Idaho Balsam Fir, Lemongrass, Palo Santo, Copaiba, Wintergreen, Helichrysum, Frankincense
- Sulfurzyme, BLM, NingXia Red, Omega Blue

Secondary Recommendations:
- PanAway, Ortho Sport, Ortho Ease, Regenolone, Marjoram, Deep Relief Roll On, Kitty Raindrop Technique Solution (with added oils)

My favorite way to start with these cases is to provide them with all of joint benefitting supplements, Copaiba orally, and a joint rub to apply to their knees once or twice a day. When Buddy came to be fostered in our home, he had injuries to his cruciate ligaments in BOTH rear legs. For him, it was likely that these injuries were nutritionally based. He was riddled with parasites, was very skinny, and his black hair actually looked brown. I realized by accident how wonderful the Kitty Raindrop Technique solution was for this condition.

He had come to our home, and I was very busy and didn't have much time to treat him that day. I just so happened to have a bottle of Kitty Raindrop solution "laying around". I decided to give him a small Raindrop Technique with it, and then was also drawn to put a puddle in my hand, and rub this onto each knee. This little guy REALLY loved the oils and proceeded to lick up the Raindrop Oils from my hand. I let him do this as well, as I felt he needed it. He probably consumed about 30 drops of the solution before he stopped. We noticed within about an hour, that he was noticeably walking better, with less favoring of his worst leg (the left rear leg).

General Directions:

Copaiba: Generally this oil will be given in larger amounts when the injury is new, and there is more discomfort. Adjust the dosage down as indicated. Generally I start by giving this oil in the food, or directly into the mouth.
    Small Dog: Dilute 1 drop with 2 drops V6. Give 1 drop twice a day.
    Medium Dog: Dilute 1 drop with 1 drop V6. Give 1 drop twice a day
    Large Dog: Give 1 neat drop twice a day.

See the supplement section for dosing information on the supplements. BLM Capsules should be given at double to triple the maintenance dose for the first 6-8 weeks in this injury. Also, Sulfurzyme should be used in increased dosages if needed. I personally give all of the supplements within the First Recommendations, then add one of the following Rub Recipes – and apply this to the knees once or twice a day, gradually increasing the amount of time between applications as indicated.

Knee Rub #1:
    In a 1 ounce glass oil bottle, add 5 drops each of Idaho Balsam Fir, Lemongrass, Palo Santo, Wintergreen, Helichrysum, Copaiba, Frankincense, and Marjoram. Fill the rest of the bottle with V6. Mix well. Drip and rub into the knee area once or twice a day for at least 1-2 weeks. Dilute further, or apply less often, if skin irritation is noted.

Knee Rub #2 – Kitty Raindrop Knee Rub:
   In a 1 ounce glass oil bottle, add 4 drops each of Oregano, Thyme, Basil, Cypress, Wintergreen, Marjoram, Peppermint, Copaiba, Helichrysum, Palo Santo or Lemongrass, and Idaho Balsam Fir. Fill the rest of the bottle with V6. Mix Well. Drip and rub onto knee area once or twice a day for at least 1-2 weeks. Dilute further, or apply less often, if skin irritation is noted.

Allergies

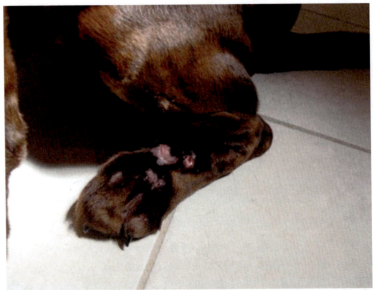

"Jack" – Food related allergies with secondary yeast and bacterial infections

Allergies are a very complicated subject, and often need a full holistic health consult to fully evaluate the causes that lie behind them. Diet is often a large part of the cause, and even in high quality foods, hidden "healthy" ingredients such as eggs could be contributing to the allergic response.

Household cleaners and common toxins have also been found to be causing the symptoms of allergies. Changing household cleaners and products to equivalent Young Living products, not only eliminates harmful chemicals, but provides more exposure to beneficial therapeutic essential oils on a daily basis.

General recommendations are made here.

First Recommendations:
- Diffuse: Clove, Thieves, or Lavender.
- Anti-Histamine Oils orally, topically, and/or diffused: Melissa, Ocotea, Basil, Lavender
- Anti-Inflammatory (steroid alternative): Raindrop Technique

- Nutritional Supplements: Allerzyme, NingXia Red, Omega Blue, Sulfurzyme, Life 5
- Other: Animal Scents Shampoo, Thieves Household Cleaner

<u>Secondary Recommendations</u>:
- Polyzyme, Mightyzyme, Detoxzyme, Digest + Cleanse, Inner Defense

<u>General Recommendations</u>: Give an Allerzyme digestive enzyme with every meal. For Large dogs, 2 or more capsules may be necessary. Give NingXia Red, and add 1-2 drops of Lavender essential oil to it. This can be given straight, or mixed into food.

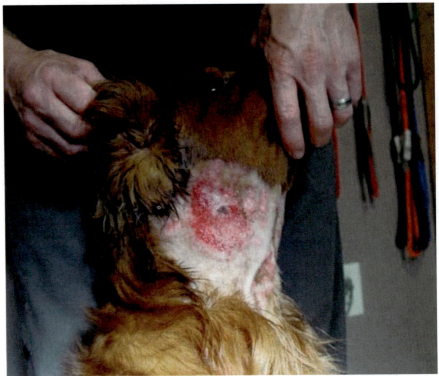
A severe "hot spot" in a dog – this one has already been shaved.

Hot Spots

A hot spot (also called pyotraumatic dermatitis and acute moist dermatitis) is a localized area of acute inflammation and exudation (pus) in the skin that is traumatized by licking, scratching, or rubbing. Bacterial overgrowth occurs on the skin, and often results in a hairless area that is moist, red and quite painful.

There is no single cause of a hot spot, but rather multiple factors that predispose to its development. Some of these factors include: inflammation resulting from allergic conditions (such as allergies, contact dermatitis, flea bites, and other parasite hypersensitivities); skin damage due to continued wetting or accumulation of moisture under a thick coat; trauma due to abrasions, foreign bodies in the coat, or irritation from clipper blades; and primary irritants contacting the skin. Moisture and weeping fluids from the inflammatory process creates a favorable climate for bacterial overgrowth and infection of the skin.

Lesions are noted more frequently during hot, humid weather. Animals are often presented to the veterinarian because they are licking or scratching a particular area, which can vary in size. The areas most commonly involved are the back and sides and the area around the head and ears. Affected skin is red, moist and in most cases weeping pus. The typical lesion will be missing hair. However, hair may still cover the lesion if it is detected early or if it is in a location that is difficult to lick or scratch. Excoriations are occasionally present due to licking or scratching.

Veterinarians make a diagnosis based on clinical appearance of lesions and a history of predisposing factors. Impression smears may be appropriate for determination of the number and type of bacteria, and a skin biopsy would be appropriate if your veterinarian suspects certain skin diseases.

Treatment of hot spots may involve sedation if the lesions are painful or the animal is fractious. Any remaining hair should be clipped from the affected area and the lesion should be cleaned with a medicated wash. Thieves Household Cleaner or Animal Scents Shampoo can be used to wash the lesion, and can be diluted if needed for very sensitive lesions. Rinse well.

Prevention of Hot Spots is not 100% but some things can be helpful. By treating allergies, ear infections, oily skin, tight collars, and many other conditions that affect the skin, we can reduce the occurrence of hot spots. Some helpful treatments include; weekly shampooing with Animal Scents Shampoo, treatment of ear infections, shaving off matts, treatment of mild skin infections, and consulting with a holistic veterinarian to find other underlying causes.

Skin Spray

Post Clipping Irritation, Hot Spots, Skin Infections, Bug Bites and more can be nicely "quieted" with this effective spray.

In a 2 ounce glass spray bottle add:

4 drops of Copaiba Essential Oil
7 drops of Lavendula angustifolia (Lavender) Essential Oil
5 drops of Melaleuca alternifolia (Tea Tree) Essential Oil
Fill the rest of the bottle with Distilled Water.

Shake well and apply to skin as needed. Generally 1-2 times a day is adequate.

Kennel Cough

Kennel cough is a very irritating, contagious cough. It can have bacterial or viral causes, and will most commonly occur after exposure to other dogs, although humans have "carried" kennel cough to other dogs after handling a contagious dog. The most effective way that I have dealt with kennel cough is to diffuse directly into an enclosed kennel with an ultrasonic diffuser. An air diffuser can be much more therapeutic, however it can be a little intense to be used in an enclosed situation as pictured below – so monitor your dog for comfort.

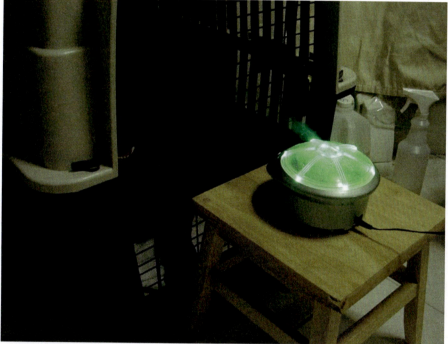
A dog getting a diffusion treatment

First Recommendations: Diffuse into an enclosed area with an ultrasonic diffuser at least 20 minutes, three times a day. Adjust times based on dog's response to the diffusion. Severe cases may benefit from having the diffuser run continuously. I adjust this according to the individual needs of the dog.

<u>Diffusion Recipe #1</u>: 4-8 drops Purification, 2 drops Eucalyptus Blue, 2 drops Copaiba

<u>Diffusion Recipe #2</u>: 4 drops Thieves, 2 drops Eucalyptus Blue, 2 drops Copaiba

<u>Diffusion Recipe #3</u>: 4-8 drops Purification or Thieves, 2 drops Frankincense or Cedarwood, 2 drops Eucalyptus Blue, 2 drops Copaiba

You may find that some dogs need less or more drops, less or more time, and less or more frequent diffusion sessions. I have not encountered a problem when diffusing for longer than 20 minutes at a time – when this has been needed for a health concern. The recommendation of limiting the amount of time we diffuse oils for, seems to be a generality for "most people" – and in our home we happily diffuse 24 hours a day for humans and pets, with no ill feelings.

<u>Secondary Diffusion Recommendations</u>: Thieves, Eucalyptus Blue, Purification, Cedarwood, Frankincense, RC, Raven, Melrose

<u>Nutritional Supplements</u>: Supporting a good immune system is important when fighting an illness.
<u>First Recommendations</u>: NingXia Red, Multigreens, Omega Blue
<u>Other Recommendations</u>: ImmuPro, True Source, Longevity, Inner Defense

Diarrhea

Sometimes it is important to know the cause of the diarrhea to know which remedies will be most effective. However, this can be difficult at times.

First you should usually start with a fast for your dog. Generally no food for 24 hours is needed to get diarrhea to stop, and for the gut to rest. Always do this with the advice of your veterinarian. Small dogs and puppies may be prone to hypoglycemia during fasting, and certain diarrhea conditions may predispose animals to more severe illness.

If your dog just got into the garbage – and you "know" the diarrhea is on its way. The most effective thing I have done is to give a dose of Inner Defense. There is a popular veterinary product on the market right now – that even mainstream veterinarians are raving about. It is a diarrhea gel that is to be given orally when situations may give a pet bacterial diarrhea. Situations this company lists are; diet and/or water changes, indiscretions in diet, environment changes, and stress. This diarrhea gel contains Carvacrol, Eugenol, Thymol, Cinnamaldehyde, Chamazulene, and Sesquiterpenoids in its active ingredients. Hmmm, sounds incredibly like the ingredients in Essential Oils!

First Recommendations: Di-Gize, Inner Defense, Life 5

General Recommendations: Apply several drops of Di-Gize to the belly. Generally neat, although monitor the area and apply V6 if any irritation is noted. Sometimes the skin will not look irritated, but the animal is obviously agitated with the site – apply V6 in these situations as well. You may also apply several drops to the feet. In severe cases, dripping the Di-Gize directly into the mouth has been very effective. Alternatively, Di-Gize can be placed into a capsule and given orally.

Small Dog: 3-10 drops Di-Gize – applied topically to belly, on feet, or into mouth or by capsule. This can be repeated up to 2-6 times a day. Monitor for skin irritation – and dilute future applications if needed.

Medium Dog: 5-15 drops Di-Gize.

Large Dog: 5-20 drops Di-Gize.

With Inner Defense – I generally just give one capsule. I will generally give this in the morning, during the fast. Then at night, I will give Life 5. Most of the time with diarrhea, I find one dose of Inner Defense is adequate. Follow the dose recommendations for Life 5, and continue this for at least 1 week with a diarrhea episode. You can give more Inner Defense if the diarrhea responds well to it, but seems to return when the Inner Defense wears off.

Horses:

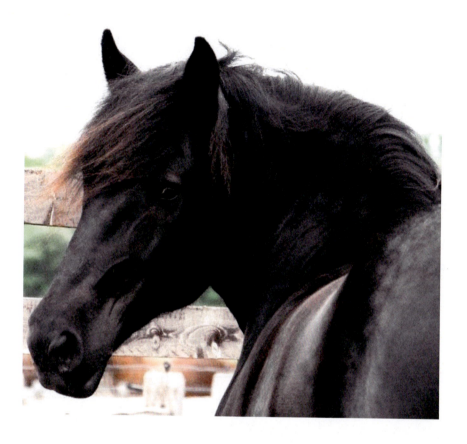

Horses respond exceptionally well to essential oils. Although they are large, they often will respond greatly to even small amounts of essential oils. My belief is that "in the wild", all animals, but especially horses, would roam and find plants that contain beneficial essential oils that they would need. Chewing and stripping bark from trees, rolling in certain plants, smelling plants while grazing, and even standing and walking through certain aromatic plants – would all expose a horse to Nature's wonderful plant oils.

Colic

The word can strike fear into the heart of any horse owner. If your horse is colicking, call a veterinarian and then grab your oils. With this protocol, many vets have been left wondering why you called by the time they have arrived at the farm.

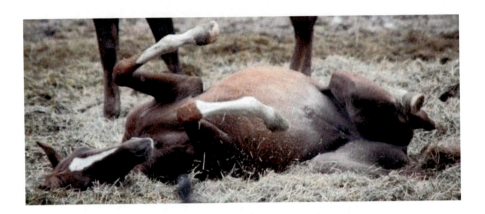

First Recommendations:
- Give 20 drops of Di-Gize and 20 drops of Peppermint dripping the oils directly into the mouth or lip. Then apply 20 drops of Di-Gize and 20 drops of Peppermint to the umbilical area (abdomen). If the horse is still colicking in 20-30 minutes, repeat both applications. If after 60 minutes, the horse is still symptomatic – it is likely to need surgery.
- At the same time apply 10-12 drops of RutaVala onto the abdomen. Also apply 3 drops of RutaVala onto the nose for calming and to help with pain.

Secondary Recommendations:
- In difficult cases of colic mix 20 drops of Di-Gize, 20 drops of Peppermint and 6-10 Detoxzyme Capsules into 4 cups of warm water. This solution can be inserted rectally and/or orally every 15 minutes for 4 doses. A "dedicated" Turkey Baster or large syringe can be used for the rectal enema, and please use a different baster/syringe for giving the solution orally. Even if you only have one or two ingredients – please use what you have on hand! Often

times this remedy will result in some pretty prominent diarrhea and flushing of the gastrointestinal system.

Di-Gize is also used to help clear anesthesia if surgery was needed.

Laminitis (aka Founder)

Many horses and ponies are prone to developing Laminitis. Many medical conditions can cause this predisposition, and it is important to work with a qualified equine veterinarian to rule out any problems that may be encouraging your horse to founder. Diet changes are key, as well as finding a great farrier who can trim your horse's hooves to benefit them the most.

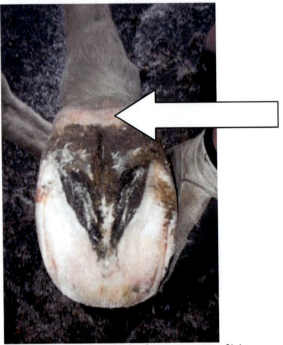

A great location to apply oils for lameness conditions

First Recommendations:
- Topically: Ortho Sport, Lemongrass, Cypress, Wintergreen, Copaiba, PanAway, Idaho Balsam Fir – rub onto legs and hooves once to twice a day as indicated by response. The amount of drops to apply, and whether they need to be diluted or not, will need to be determined for the individual animal. I typically will start with undiluted oils – between 2-10 drops onto each leg, around the coronet, and especially focusing on the area shown in the picture above. This is typically the location that you will feel "pulses" in cases of laminitis.

- When deciding on which oils to use for Laminitis – I try to make sure I have some main areas covered: an oil to increase circulation (Cypress), an oil to decrease inflammation (Copaiba, Wintergreen, PanAway, Idaho Balsam Fir), and oils to address the main cause of the laminitis occurrence. For example – a pony getting into the grain would get DiGize as well.
- Raindrop Technique – daily to weekly as indicated by the severity of the case. I will typically start with a standard Raindrop Technique, and then evaluate how the horse does from that one application. Adding other oils into the technique is fine. In cases of Laminitis – I will most certainly make sure that oils are applied to the feet and hooves during the Raindrop application – sometimes in higher quantities than usual.
- DiGize orally – 5-10 drops once to twice a day.

<u>Secondary Recommendations</u>: Ortho Ease, NingXia Red, Clove Oil Orally

Any of the oils can be applied topically or orally. In severe cases, I may try oral along with the topical applications. Generally, I will start with 5-10 drops of an oil orally, and monitor for response. If I see an improvement, I will see how long it lasts for. If the effects wear off in 3 hours, I will try to increase the dose or give the oils every 2 hours. There is no right or wrong, and it is important to see how the horse does, and adjust from there. Do not continue a regimen that is not helping or is causing distress to a horse. There are plenty of other oils to try, and if you don't see positive effects within 24 hours, try something else!

Strangles

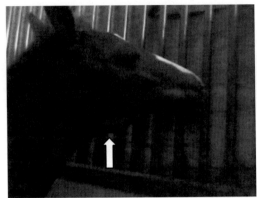

An abscess under the throat-latch of a foal. This abscess was restricting breathing, and the foal would extend his head upward, and puff his cheeks.

One of the worst horse germs out there is Streptococcus equi – the bacteria that causes Strangles. The disease is called Strangles, because enormous abscesses are formed – which literally can "strangle" a horse to death. The bacteria can live in the environment for months. It can be transmitted on shoes, hands, clothing, tack, and of course on other horses. Nothing is safe – the wood inside of a stall, feed troughs, transport trailers, and even dirt can harbor the bacteria for a very, very long time.

For prevention, each horse entering a new farm should get a Raindrop Technique. If possible, every existing horse already on the farm would get a Raindrop prior to the new horse's arrival as well. At least one week before the "exposure".

For horses that travel and show, performing a Raindrop Technique on them at least one week prior to the show or event is recommended. If the horse in question is not sensitive to the Raindrop Technique and it's detoxifying actions – then doing this Raindrop the night before would be great. Welts are the most common symptom seen from the aggressive detoxifying effects of a Raindrop. I see this most commonly in horses with health concerns or that have been overly vaccinated. See the section on Raindrop Technique for Horses for more information.

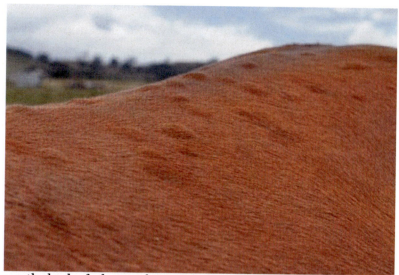
Welts on the back of a horse after a Raindrop Technique – discussed further on page 107

Horses "at risk" for Strangles would benefit from regular Raindrop Technique – at least monthly. These would be horses who live on a farm with show horses, participate in outside equine activities, and really any horse that would be exposed to another horse in any way shape or form; even being transported in someone else's trailer.

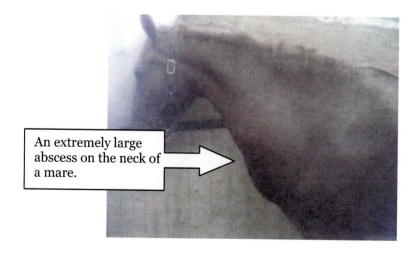
An extremely large abscess on the neck of a mare.

It is ideal if every new horse would be quarantined for at least 30 days prior to being "released" into the herd. This may not always be feasible, but it is the best way to make sure that all forms of bacteria, viruses, and parasites are not passed onto other horses. In areas where new horses are being quarantined diffusing Thieves Oil with an air diffuser would be ideal. Monitor the horse for how long the diffuser can be run, and how often. Again, the more "toxic" the horse, or the more health problems they have – the less amount of time they can tolerate diffusion. We had one horse that lathered up within 10 minutes of diffusing Thieves near his stall. We still diffused, but with more ventilation, and for shorter amounts of time – more frequently. Eventually, he could tolerate more and more.

In situations where it is not urgent to diffuse a "heavy hitting oil" – then picking a more mild oil to diffuse such as Lemon or Purification – may be a good choice. However, with this stallion – we were trying to prevent the spread of Strangles – so we stayed with the Thieves Oil.

Thieves Household Cleaner should be used in all areas around the quarantine area, and to disinfect a farm with an outbreak. To "clean" one farm, we added Thieves Household Cleaner to the Arena Sprayer and sprayed the paddocks, arena, walk ways – anywhere there could by hiding bacteria. We also used the cleaner in the foot baths, to wash out clothes, spray the bottoms of our shoes, and even the door handles on our truck. We would rub Thieves Oil onto our hands between paddocks if we weren't able to wash our hands.

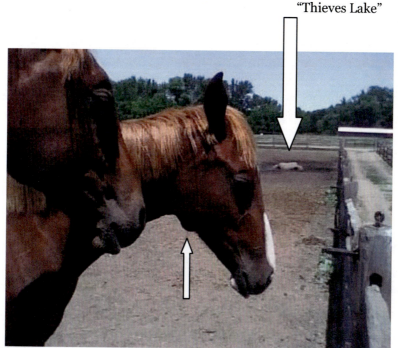

The large puddle that was treated with Thieves Oil – slightly dried up. You can see a swollen lymph node under the throat of this yearling – the start of Strangles.

At this same farm, there was a large puddle in a paddock full of yearlings. Some of these yearlings had proven very difficult to catch and to treat. We were relying on the fact that since the majority of the horses had gotten a Raindrop Technique, that they would act as giant "horse diffusers" and spread the benefits to the horses we couldn't catch. Being young and silly horses, we often saw them playing in a large puddle during our futile attempts to catch them. As they needed oils, one way or another, I dumped an entire bottle of Thieves essential oil into the puddle. As they stood, pawed and played in the puddle – they now had "aromatherapy" and didn't even know it! The oils on the surface of the puddle almost certainly clung to their feet and legs, and were absorbed readily. Treating them, when they didn't even know it!

As we were applying the Raindrop Technique to several of the Strangles horses, it "felt" right to also apply each Raindrop oil to large abscesses that had refused to break open and drain. Within a day or two – we literally saw abscesses explode and drain easily. I thought one of the farm workers was going to pass out when a large ball of pus actually "shot" out of an abscess and across the stall after an application! Remember, it is okay to experiment with different things. No one will take you to "Essential Oil Jail" if you apply oils differently than someone else. We have even applied the Raindrop oils to leg infections, joints, and other locations when needed, and have seen great success.

First Recommendations:
- Raindrop Technique – daily.
- <u>Oral Oils</u>: Ravensara, Exodus II, Thieves, Cinnamon, Oregano, Longevity, ImmuPower – once or twice a day or more.
- <u>Topical Oils</u>: Ravensara, Exodus II, Thieves, Cinnamon, Oregano, Longevity, ImmuPower – daily
- <u>Diffuse</u>: Thieves, Ravensara – as often and as long as possible.
- <u>Thieves Household Cleaner</u> – Arena Sprayers, Foot Baths, Tack Wash, Disinfectants...

Secondary Recommendations:
- DiGize Orally, Lemongrass Diffused

General Recommendations:
- Everyone always wants to know how many drops to start with. Truly, this often has to be evaluated for each individual horse – seeing what they will tolerate and how they respond. With oral oils, I often start with 5-10 drops of Exodus II and Ravensara, twice a day. Then if DiGize and ImmuPower can also be given, I will add this into the oral regimen as well. This amount may increase if a horse seems to really crave a certain oil. Generally, the body will do better with smaller amounts of oils, given more frequently. If this is a possibility in the owner's schedule, then I will give oils 4-6 times a day.

- With topical application, oils may be inserted into the Raindrop Technique, or even applied in "Raindrop Fashion" up the back without the full Raindrop Technique. See the section on Raindrop Technique for Horses, for more in-depth information about monitoring skin and adjusting the technique for sensitive horses. In the case of Strangles, it is such a serious disease, that even in the presence of welts and slight skin irritation, I generally continue to apply the Raindrop Technique daily. With Strangles, I would generally start with 6-8 drops of each Raindrop Oil during the application. When adding oils into the Raindrop Technique – I generally only add between 1-3 of the additional topical oils recommended. 6-8 drops of the additional oil is also usually applied.

- When using oils topically – you can start with a few drops of the oil and see if dilution is needed. If the horse does not appear agitated or the skin is not inflamed, you can add additional drops after about 10 minutes.

- Locations to apply: Sometimes you can only apply the oils where the horse will allow you to. So if this means dumping them into a puddle, or adding some to water (make sure the horse still drinks) – then this is what we have to do. If the horse becomes dangerous to handle while trying to apply oils to the feet or the back – by all means – DO NOT APPLY THEM! Your safety is the most important thing. I have even heard of people "throwing" oils at a pony that they could not get near – and still saw amazing benefits. Sometimes, we can only do what we can – so if the recommended way isn't working – do not be afraid to "blaze your own trail"!

- With Strangles, it is likely that you will not see major results within 24 hours. However, I generally like to see "something" within 24 hours, that tells me that our chosen remedies are being effective. This may even mean that things just didn't "get worse" – especially in a horse that was continuing to decline every day. If you aren't seeing some sort of positive effect from your chosen regimen – change things!

Thrush

Thrush is a bacterial infection of the hoof, caused by an anaerobic bacteria (this means the bacteria does not like oxygen). It can become a painful condition, and affect the frog of the hoof severely if left unattended. Thankfully, essential oils are incredibly oxygenating, and can penetrate tissues exceptionally well. My own farrier has been amazed at how quickly thrush is resolving now that she uses Thieves Essential Oil on her cases. She still trims away nasty tissue, and tries to provide a clean environment for the hoof, but she has seen amazing strides in treatment from simply dripping Thieves Oil on the underside of the hoof – neat. This is generally applied once to twice a day – with enough drops to coat the area. We have not seen "over-application" at all with regards to thrush, but monitoring sensitive tissues is still a good idea. For cases with severe financial restrictions – we have even diluted the Thieves oil in V6, and still seen wonderful results.

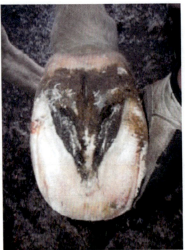

Apply oils to the entire underside of the hoof

First Recommendations:
- Thieves Essential Oil applied neat to the underside of the hoof and frog. 5-10 or more drops, applied to each hoof, once or twice a day – or as needed to control symptoms.

Secondary Recommendations:
- Australian Blue, Melrose, Oregano, Longevity, Cinnamon, Clove – applied topically
- Thieves Household Cleaner – scrub the underside of the hoof well. Alternatively – create a foot soak with the Thieves Household Cleaner.
- Raindrop Technique – this may be very helpful for a horse with more severe symptoms. Dripping each of the Raindrop Oils on the underside of the hoof would be a great idea!

Navicular Disease (Syndrome)

Equine specialists have still not figured out a direct cause or treatment for Navicular Disease. In general, it is believed to be a result of long bars and heels on the horse's hoof – which causes inflammation around the Navicular bone resulting in sometimes severe lameness. It seems that the congestion of the digital arteries result in more pain than the damage to the Navicular bone itself – which is often noticed most on x-rays. Recent studies have proven that there is no direct correlation between the shape of the cavities within the Navicular bone and clinical lameness.

Removing shoes and working with more natural living conditions have returned many horses back to a functional hoof physiology. Although this process can take many months.

In general this condition is noted to have heel pain, however horses may stand in various positions to escape the painful portion of the foot. Symptoms and severity seem to vary with each horse as there is no "one" cause of Navicular Syndrome. It often feels like a losing battle –and consulting with an excellent barefoot farrier is of the utmost importance. Getting references and asking if they have successfully dealt with Navicular disease is very important.

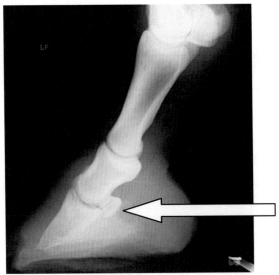

The Navicular Bone

First Recommendations:
- Raindrop Technique – as often as needed, also applied to the coronet, frog and bulb areas.
- Oral Oils: Clove (lot's of this oil), Copaiba, DiGize
- Topical Oils: Clove, Copaiba, Lemongrass, Cypress
- Sulfurzyme, NingXia Red, BLM
- Consult an equine nutritionist for dietary recommendations – NO sweet feed!

Secondary Recommendations:
- Topical Oils: PanAway, Idaho Balsam Fir, Wintergreen, Helichrysum, Spruce

General Recommendations: This may vary with how severe the horse's lameness is. When needed, Raindrop application daily may be necessary – and should especially be applied to the feet/legs. Oral oils may need to be given 4-6 times a day in times of severe pain. With Clove Oil – you could start with 5-10 drops twice a day orally, and monitor for response. Increasing the amount or the frequency can be tried if no benefit is noticed. Some horses have gotten up to 20 drops at a time, multiple times a day for severe lameness flare ups.

DiGize and Copaiba can also be started orally with 5-10 drops 2-6 times a day. Monitor the individual horse to see what comfort they achieve, and adjust timing and frequency from there. Many horses take these oils orally very easily. I have just dripped them into the bottom lip of my pony with very little if any protest. Although, sometimes a curled lip afterward!

White Line Disease (Seedy Toe)

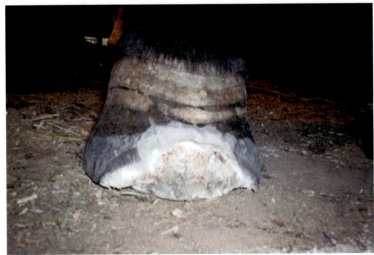

A fairly severe case of White Line Disease – with a hoof wall resection

My own pony always had some evidence of "separation" at each trim, after all, this is why we got her. She was lame and the owners were moving. What a better new home than with a veterinarian! At one particular trim our farrier noted White Line Disease (WLD), which is thought to be a fungal infection between the layers of the hoof wall. My pony was going to need a large amount of hoof "resected" or cut away – according to the traditional treatment for WLD. As a holistic veterinarian, cutting away large portions of a horse's hoof does not seem like a good idea – so I only allowed my farrier to carve a small channel into the hoof wall. Knowing that the cause of the WLD may be fungal, but could have other origins as well – I decided to put Thieves Essential Oil into the channel twice a day. I put between 3-5 drops into the groove, and also onto each surface of every other hoof. It was amazing how the hoof wall "sucked" up the oil, and you could actually see the penetration into the tissues.

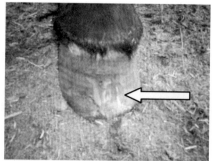
Shadow's very small groove in the hoof wall – barely detectable.

Two and a half weeks later, my farrier returned for a recheck. Not only was the WLD gone, but she had never seen such a fast resolution of it. AND, it also appeared that the chronic separation and slight laminitis that she had always shown in her hooves was gone! My farrier actually asked if I had cut the feet off of another pony and transplanted them onto mine! I feel that the Thieves Oil brought in oxygenation, decreased inflammation, increased circulation, and killed the fungal infection – leading to her miraculous recovery. To this day, she has never shown a recurrence of the previous separation in the hoof wall – which had been present for 3 years prior to the Thieves oil being applied.

First Recommendations:
- Thieves Oil – topically onto hoof, or into hoof resection. 3-10 drops twice a day until resolved.

Secondary Recommendations:
- Melrose, Longevity, Oregano, Lemongrass, Australian Blue, Wintergreen, Cypress

Other oils can be applied in a similar amount and fashion to the hooves.

Rain Rot

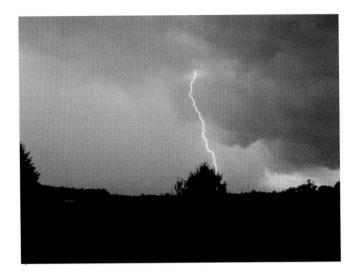

Rain Rot is a bacterial infection of the skin, mainly caused by excessive moisture. Fungal infections can look very similar, and it is important to recognize that not all Rain Rot may be bacterial in origin. Maintaining dry skin is very important to the healing process.

First Recommendations:
- Shampoo the affected area with Thieves Household Cleaner. Rinse well. Make sure the area can dry well.
- Shampoo the affected area with Animal Scents Shampoo.
- Additional oils may be added to either wash solution – to make it more powerful. 5-10 drops added to a tablespoon or more of wash is a starting point.
- Topical Oils: Melrose, Purification, Thieves, Longevity – for antibacterial and antifungal benefits.
- Topical Oils: Lavender, Patchouli – for soothing benefits.

Secondary Recommendations:
- Raindrop Technique – this may be difficult to perform on severely irritated skin, however will have great immune benefits as well as antibacterial action.
- Supporting good nutrition will help with healing – Sulfurzyme, NingXia Red, Longevity Oil orally.

Raindrop Technique for Horses

The Raindrop Technique is indicated for almost any condition. There are seven main oils within a standard Raindrop Technique, and when you think about all of the properties that these oils possess – it is hard to find a living being that *wouldn't* benefit from a Raindrop!

- Oregano: anti-aging, powerful anti-viral, antibacterial, antifungal, antiparasitic, anti-inflammatory, immune stimulant
- Thyme: anti-aging, highly anti-microbial, antifungal, antiviral, antiparasitic.
- Basil: Anti-spasmodic, antiviral, antibacterial, anti-inflammatory, muscle relaxant, anti-histamine
- Cypress: Improves circulation, strengthens capillaries, anti-infectious, anti-spasmodic, discourages fluid retention
- Wintergreen: Anticoagulant, antispasmodic, highly anti-inflammatory, vasodilator, analgesic/anesthetic, reduces blood pressure, all types of pain, musculoskeletal problems.
- Marjoram: Muscle soothing, relieve body and joint discomfort, soothe digestive tract, antibacterial, antifungal, vasodilator, lowers blood pressure, promotes intestinal peristalsis, expectorant, mucolytic
- Peppermint: Driving Oil. Anti-inflammatory, antitumoral, antiparasitic (worms), antibacterial, antiviral, antifungal, gall bladder/digestive stimulant, pain-relieving.

There are as many ways to give a Raindrop Technique, as there are people using Essential Oils! Here is a method for a "down and dirty" Raindrop application, that gets the oils on the horse quickly and effectively. I have found that when using essential oils for health concerns in my veterinary patients, that if I required the owner to do a procedure that took 40-60 minutes per day to perform – that it was unlikely to get done. If you have the time, and you want to enjoy the full process of a Raindrop Technique with your horse – by all means – please complete the entire process. There are many references available that demonstrate giving a Raindrop Technique. Make sure to sign up for future newsletters on my website at www.OilyVet.com or www.CrowRiverAnimalHospital.com, to keep up to date on the arrivals of new DVD's demonstrating all sorts of oil applications – including Raindrop Technique.

The most important thing to remember is that ANY oils are better than no oils at all. So, if you are pressed for time – your horse will benefit more from just getting sprinkled with oils, than not having any applied at all. I find that so many people feel that if they do it wrong – they will somehow go to "Raindrop Jail" or scar their horse for life! WRONG! Relax and let your horse show you that even standing in a puddle with oils floating on top of the surface – can in fact be beneficial!

So, just what IS a Raindrop Technique?

A Raindrop Technique is a special way of applying several (often 7-9) different oils topically over the spinal area. This technique was created by the founder of Young Living, Gary Young. The technique he created combined the therapeutic use of essential oils with several ancient modalities; from Native American rituals to Tibetan Reflexology. This technique was originally designed for humans, and then has been adapted for use in the animal kingdom. There is a Raindrop Technique Kit available from Young Living, and this includes an instructional DVD for humans within it. This DVD is helpful to watch, so that you can have an understanding of the procedure we are trying to emulate for an animal.

In the application, the chosen oils are dripped from tail to head, from a distance of about 3-6 inches from the spine. Combined with specialized strokes and reflexology techniques (called VitaFlex), Raindrop Technique can be a powerful tool that anyone can use.

To perform a Raindrop on a horse that has never had one before – I may start out conservatively and use less drops of each oil. However, in a horse with a severe medical concern – using the full amounts of oils may be needed. Some horses may also "show" that they need fewer drops of oils applied or pre-diluted oils applied to them. The most common reason for this adjustment is for horses that "welt" from the application of oils.

There are several reasons why the welts may appear. Generally, I find the welts to occur in horses that are more "toxic" in general. They usually have more health concerns, have been on traditional medications, or are typically "over" vaccinated. Most horses will gradually welt less and less as the detoxification occurs. Over time, it is found that these same horses that welted severely when first getting a Raindrop, will not welt in the future. However, this may take many months of exposure to essential oils to completely detoxify them.

There are several schools of thought about what to do when a horse welts from a Raindrop. For me, it depends on the severity of the health concern – for how I will exactly proceed. If it is a life threatening situation, as in Strangles, then I will continue to give the Raindrop Technique daily if needed – even applying the full amount of drops. However, I will dilute the area with V6 after the application of neat oils to make it more comfortable for the horse. Some horses are not uncomfortable at all with the welts, and may not need the V6 applied. Other horses have rolled on the ground with irritation. Creating this level of irritation in any animal is never warranted. Diluting the oils before application, applying less oils at a time, applying V6 after neat application, or even omitting certain oils from the Raindrop Technique is just fine.

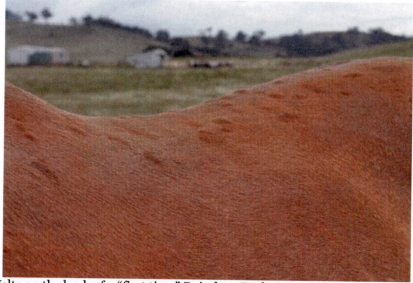

Welts on the back of a "first time" Raindrop Technique recipient. This horse has multiple health concerns.

Another horse owner I know was giving her horse a Raindrop application for a lameness issue. The horse had Raindrop applications previously, and had not welted. However, with this health condition – he proceeded to welt severely from the same exact technique. In this owner's eyes, this was a good sign of things being "cleared up". She continued to perform the Raindrop daily for this horse, and chose to aggressively deal with the problem. As a result, his lameness resolved in record time – at the same time that the welts stopped occurring!

Sometimes oils can be given orally instead of topically for severe cases. Any exposure to essential oils can help "detox" an animal – so changing the route of administration can make gradual detoxification more comfortable. Diffusing oils, adding oils to drinking water, applying "gentle" oils topically, or giving oils orally or in foods can aid in a slower more comfortable detox.

DiGize and Longevity are often oils chosen to give orally to horses that welt up. Giving 5-10 drops of each oil – DiGize in the morning and Longevity at night – can aid a horse.

Other oils have anti-histamine activity, and can be given orally to horses that are irritated with their welts. Melissa, Ocotea, and Basil oils have anti-histamine activity. Starting with 3-5 drops orally and evaluating the response is a good starting point. The number of drops given can certainly be increased as well. Mixing more expensive oils like Melissa with an equal amount of Copaiba (a magnifier oil) – can reduce the amount of oil that must be given. Copaiba is also very anti-inflammatory – so can add its own benefits into the regimen.

The Basic "Animal Hospital" Raindrop Technique (without hoof application):

Please watch the DVD within the Raindrop Technique Kit – this will help you understand the various steps. The following steps are for a regular sized horse – so you may want to scale down the amount of drops for a small pony, miniature horse, or foal.

- Place 3-6 drops of **Valor** into both hands. Balance your horse with your hands behind the ears on the top of the neck. Stand in a safe location of course, and always be mindful that you are working on a large animal, that could injure you. For horses that do not tolerate this, you can balance at the withers as well. For horses that seem to need more balancing or really enjoy the Valor oil, balancing at the poll and at the withers is just fine as well. With severe time constraints or with animals that will not allow balancing of any sort – omit the balancing steps.

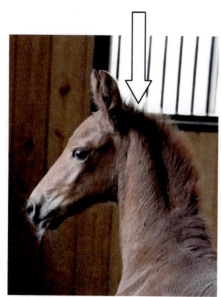
The Poll

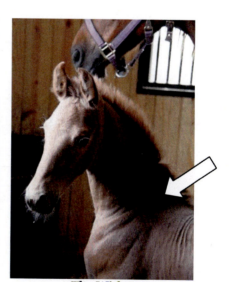
The Withers

- Place 3-6 drops of **Valor** into both hands. Balance your horse with your hands over the pelvic area or sacrum.

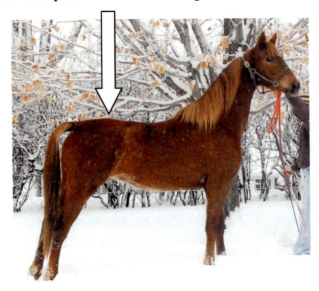

- If **Hoof Application of Oils** is desired, insert here. See description below. Hoof application is not 100% necessary, but is encouraged for any hoof or lameness concern.

- Next drip approximately 6 drops of **Oregano Oil** from the tail to the top of the neck. Generally, try to hold the bottle approximately 6 inches above the back as you drip them. This is due to the electrical field that we all have surrounding our bodies. As we drip the oils through this field, the natural frequency of the oil provides benefits to the energy field.

  Be careful not to get oils onto the face or near the eyes of the horse. As with the typical Raindrop Technique – "scratch" the oils into the back with your fingers. Alternatively, you may only be able to rub the oils into the back, with a clockwise circular action. Repeat either of these methods three times (if possible) – from tail to head. This oil is a "hot" oil, and may be an oil that you will see a horse develop discomfort from. Dilute the area with V6 if you see signs of irritation. Then, for future Raindrops, you may want to use fewer drops of Oregano, or dilute it with V6 before the application. There are some thoughts out there that diluting the oils will negate or greatly lessen the effects of the Raindrop Technique. I have not found this to be true. If horses are greatly irritated from an oil, it is less likely that the owner can give the horse a Raindrop at all, and this event will truly eliminate any benefits.

- Then, drip 6 drops of **Thyme Oil** in the same manner as the Oregano. Rubbing the oils in three times, up the back. This oil is also "hot", and is probably the most common oil that I see skin irritation and welts from. I try to stagger the "drip site" of this oil from where the Oregano Oil "fell". This way, the skin will not be getting oils applied in only one location, over and over again.

- After the application of Oregano and Thyme – I almost always apply **V6 Diluting Oil** from the tail to the head. Depending on the horse and how they appear to be tolerating the procedure, I may apply more or less V6 to the back. Rub and massage the oil into the spine area – three times is not important for this step – nor is the method of the rubbing. However, I do find that if the horse enjoys each step – this is a good way to encourage "easy" Raindrops in the future. So if there is a style of rubbing that the horse enjoys, please try to provide it!

- Next, you will apply 6 drops of **Basil Oil** in the same exact manner. Although each oil can have a different amount of drops – I find it beneficial to my horse owners to just keep each oil at the same amount of drops at first. It is much easier to remember. In the future, as you become more comfortable with "tweaking" the Raindrop, you can apply more or less of particular oils, if it was indicated for a certain condition. For example, I may apply more Basil Oil when the horse was indicating a need for an antihistamine.

- Apply the next oils the same way. 6 drops of **Cypress Oil**. This oil increases circulation, so occasionally in a sensitive horse, the increase in circulation can bring a more intense irritation to them. At any point in the Raindrop application, you can always apply more V6 whenever needed. You can also reduce the amount of oils you are applying, or even stop the Raindrop if you are concerned that the horse is not doing well. One horse I consulted on, rolled and became agitated with each additional oil application. Nasal discharge also started to flow from the nostrils. This horse obviously had some "junk" to clear out – however, if the horse does not have a life threatening illness, we can do this clearing gently. If this sort of a reaction occurs, apply V6 oil to the back, and wait until the horse is comfortable – and either stop the Raindrop or modify the future oils applied. Pre-diluting the future oils or applying fewer drops is better than getting trampled or rolled on!

- **Wintergreen Oil** is next. Apply 6 drops of this oil. Wintergreen is an anti-inflammatory oil. There are occasional animals that this appears to be a "hot" oil for – so keep this in mind.

- **Optional**: If you wanted to **Insert Other Oils** into a Raindrop Technique – this is generally the location to do it. Don't worry – if you forget and insert oils before Wintergreen or after Marjoram – you will not go to "Raindrop Jail". There has never been a Raindrop given the same way twice – and if there are people that accomplish this – they have far too much study time on their hands, and they should come over and clean my house! Usually I will not insert more than 1-3 different oils into the Raindrop Technique. However, no one will arrest you if you did!

- **Marjoram Oil** is the next oil. Apply 6-12 drops of this oil. Again, you can keep the amount at 6 drops at first for easy remembering. This oil is very good for all muscular conditions and so is generally applied on the muscles up both sides of the spine. You can continue the basic rubbing in that we did for all of the oils, but this is also a step where doing more of a muscular massage would be great. At first, it is just fine to keep all of the steps the same. I find if I give too many instructions or variations to my clients at first, they can become overwhelmed.

- **Optional: Copaiba Oil** – although not a part of the "true Raindrop" I often insert Copaiba Oil here. I know I said that I insert most other oils behind Wintergreen, but Copaiba oil is an exception for me. Since this oil is a magnifier oil, I will often apply it after almost every other oil is applied, the exception being Peppermint, which is explained below. Not only will the Copaiba Oil make every other oils' actions "stronger", it also has its own health benefits. It is the highest powered anti-inflammatory in 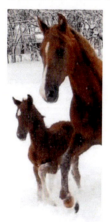 the essential oil world and also has gastro-protective properties. Something most horses will almost always benefit from. Although Copaiba magnifies the other oils, I have not found that it increases the "hotness" or welts caused by other oils. It seems that only the health benefits are amplified! For some horses, this can be an easy way to be able to use less oils, and get the same results.

- **Peppermint Oil** is "always" the last oil. It is a driving oil, which means that it will help "drive" the Copaiba and the rest of the oils deeper into the tissues. So being the last oil – just "drives the other oils home". The main reason I may omit this oil is in the dead of winter. This is a "cold" oil, so it could cause some animals to become chilled more than is comfortable for them.

- When possible, the application of oils is followed by a **Vitaflex Reflexology** procedure. This is best shown or explained by watching the Raindrop DVD, however in horses, we often use our entire hand and fingers instead of just our thumbs. See the picture sequence below to see how it is done. You will "walk" both hands up the sides of the spine, gradually inching forward after every repetition of the Vitaflex maneuver. Think of an inchworm, gradually inching its way up the back. Go from tail to head, and repeat this three times as well. If a horse will not allow this step to happen, I omit it.

Vitaflex

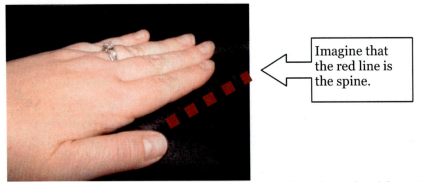

Imagine that the red line is the spine.

You would "mirror" this with your other hand on the other side of the spine. Both hands will do the action at the same time.

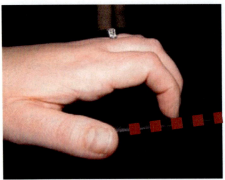

Roll your fingers up, and onto their points.

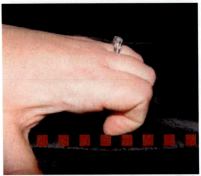 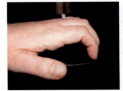 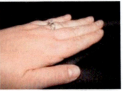

Continue rolling your fingers all the way over, onto your finger nails. Roll your hands back to the starting position, then move both hands forward ½ to 1 inch, and repeat until you have traveled all the way from the base of the tail to the poll.

Raindrop Technique – Hoof Application:

With conditions involving the hoof or lameness, or for a true "full" Raindrop Technique – applying oils to the hooves is definitely beneficial. However, when we were treating an entire horse farm for Strangles – we were not able to include the hoof application to all of the horses. After all, we administered approximately 80 Raindrops A DAY, and sometimes on fairly un-cooperative horses. Even without this step, we still saw huge benefits. Alternatively, you could also give the Hoof Application *only* when pressed for time, or when dealing with a hoof or lameness issue.

Generally, oils are applied to the hooves after the Valor balancing steps described previously. Some people apply Valor to the hooves before the "body" balancing, and some people apply the "body" balancing before applying the Valor to the hooves. I have not found it to matter either way. I tend to want to deal with the hooves all at once, so will balance the head and rump first, and then move onto the entire hoof protocol.

The rest of the "spinal" Raindrop is administered after the hooves.

- Most people start with the Right Front Hoof, and apply 3-6 drops of **Valor** to the bulb area. Then move to the Right Rear Hoof, and apply the Valor the same. Then the Left Rear Leg, and ending at the Left Front Leg. Again, if pressed for time, or when dealing with an uncooperative horse, I may omit this step, especially when the condition is not structural. However, almost any hoof issue will affect the way the horse will carry themselves, and Valor can be beneficial as the "Chiropractor in a Bottle".

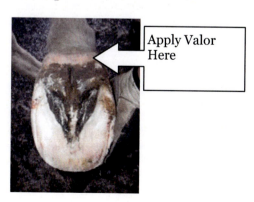

- Next you will apply the Raindrop Oils to the legs/hooves. Again there are many variations here as well. Firstly – some people only apply the "Raindrop" oils to the rear legs – I will often include the front legs in conditions that will benefit from having the oils applied near the leg and hoof. For instance if the horse is having a lameness issue in the front leg, or has an abscess in a front hoof, I am certainly going to apply the raindrop oils to the front legs as well. If all four legs are to have the oils applied, generally people also start at the Right Front Leg, and circle back to the Left Front Leg, as described for the Valor.

- Another variation would be applying Oregano, Thyme, Basil, Cypress, Wintergreen, Marjoram, and Peppermint to the first leg, then moving to the second leg and applying all of the oils, and so forth. Again, other people will apply the Oregano to the Right Front Leg, then the Right Rear Leg, then the Left Rear Leg, then the Left Front Leg – then move onto the Thyme application, etc... Again, I have not found a huge difference in benefits from choosing one way over the other, so I allow for the human to pick which way suits them best. Depending on if I have a helper or not, will often determine how I will apply the oils. If I have to grab and open each individual bottle of oil, I am more likely to play "ring around the horsey" and apply each oil one at a time.

- The other main difference is where the oils are applied on the legs. Often Oregano and Thyme are applied only to the coronet band area, as these are "hotter" oils. However, true to form, I have applied these oils to the leg area when there has been a tendon infection or a joint that would benefit from having the oils applied over the area. Many times the legs are more sensitive than the coronet band – and so dilution may be necessary.

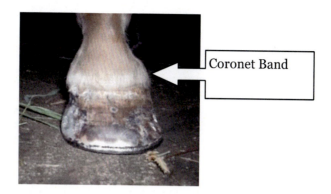

Coronet Band

- Once you have decided which feet you will be applying oils to, you will start by applying **Oregano Oil**. Generally place 3 drops into the palm of your non-dominant hand. Circle your finger tips into the oil puddle, then Vitaflex the oil into the coronet band. Do the Vitaflex the same way as shown for the spine, however you will just be using one hand. Start at the front center of the coronet band, and Vitaflex outward toward the rear of the hoof. Dip your fingers into the oil for each round of Vitaflex. Repeat this three times, on each side of the coronet band. When you move to the next leg, you will add another 3 drops of Oregano Oil to your hand, and repeat the entire procedure.

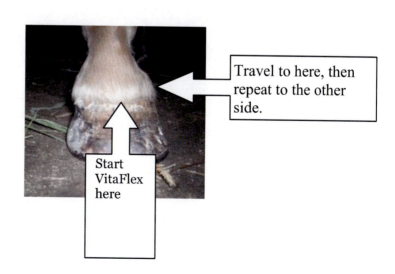

Travel to here, then repeat to the other side.

Start VitaFlex here

- Next, you will apply **Thyme Oil** to each of the chosen coronet bands.

- Depending on the condition, the next oils are generally applied to the inner surface of the rear legs, from the knee (stifle) down the leg. When indicated, you could also apply the oils to the coronet area. Again, I will let the condition decide on where the oils need to be applied, and may apply to both areas if I think it will be beneficial. If the front legs are to "receive" oils, then they can be applied to either the coronet band or to the area needing the application. Again, you will circle your finger tips into the oil, and Vitaflex the oil down the leg, three times.

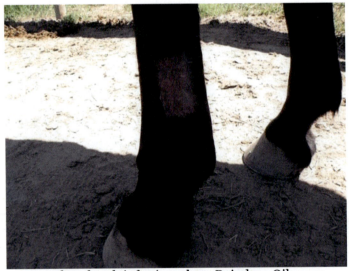

A tendon sheath infection where Raindrop Oils were applied to the area over the tendon in a front leg.

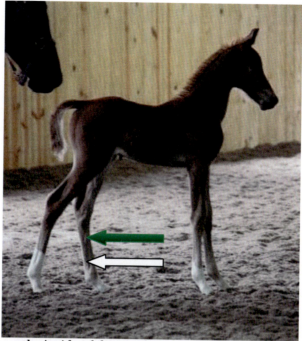

Apply oils on the inside of the rear leg, starting at the green (top) arrow, and traveling down to the white (bottom) arrow.

- The next oils that will be applied are **<u>Basil, Cypress, Wintergreen, Marjoram, and Peppermint</u>**. And, to make things more confusing, you could insert different oils as well – just as described for the "spinal" Raindrop.
- Once you have applied all of these oils to the legs and locations you have chosen – now proceed to applying the spinal portion of the Raindrop Technique.

Now you can see why I try to create as simple of a Raindrop Technique as possible for "newbies". Not only can giving a Raindrop Technique every day take up a considerable amount of time, but all of the different variations can cause some major mental stress for the owner of an already ill horse. Many will just shut down, and choose to not apply any oils at all to their horse. This is the last thing that is needed, so if a procedure needs to be simplified for the first few weeks, then that is what is best for the horse and owner.

You Never Get a Second Chance...
To Make a First Impression

None of us would feel good to have a visitor come into our home or animal facility, and say "Yuck, it sure smells like animals in here." Now of course, that is what we would expect a grooming salon, veterinary clinic, or house with animals to smell like – but it doesn't mean we have to accept it.

How wonderful I feel when people enter my veterinary clinic and home and say "Wow, it smells like a spa in here!" I needed to achieve this odor control in a natural and safe manner. I would rather have my clinic "smell like a vet clinic" than use toxic air fresheners and odor eliminators that I had documented to cause liver and kidney problems in my patients.

Area Odor Control with Cold Diffusion

The easiest way to have your home or facility smell extraordinary is to utilize a diffuser to send out essential oils into the air. There are many models of diffusers – it is important that they do not heat the essential oils as heat will damage the oil and render it less effective. All of the models of diffusers from Young Living will safely diffuse oils into the air without damaging them. I recommend that most people start with an ultrasonic diffuser – one that is run with water. These are the most flexible in their use, and can be used in many different ways.

Plant Extracts Inc. also carries a high quality diffuser that I recommend to many of my clients. You can find their diffuser at www.PlantExtractsInc.com, and you can purchase them in wholesale quantities as well. Although I do not use their essential oils currently on animals, I do love their diffuser.

It is important that diffusers be of high quality, and designed to run with high potency essential oils, as in the case with medical grade oils. Even though less expensive diffusers can be found on E-bay and other sources, I generally recommend staying with the brands that I know will not deteriorate with medical grade essential oils.

Oils and their Uses in Diffusion...

There are so many ways to use oils, but these are a few of my favorite suggestions:

- **_Purification Oil Blend_** – Primary oil for odor elimination. However I have seen astonishing medical benefits from diffusing this oil in my animal hospital: A reduction in the transmission of disease, a halt of diarrhea, fevers breaking, kennel cough decreasing drastically, and even dogs responding emotionally – calmer and less agitated.
- **_Peace and Calming_** – This oil blend provides exactly that; peace and calming. Wonderful for dogs with anxiety, separation issues, hatred of being kenneled...
- **_Christmas Spirit_** – A favorite of everyone. Cinnamon, Orange, and Spruce oils make for a classic scent. The medical grade oils do so much more.
- **_Other Suggestions:_** Harmony, Thieves, Abundance, Valor, Orange, Lemon...

Supplements and Dosing Suggestions:

BLM Capsules:

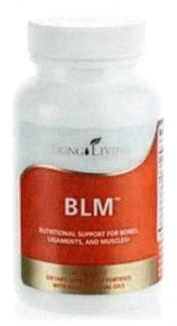

- BLM Powder contains Xylitol, the Capsules do NOT. Xylitol has been linked to toxic effects in some dogs – so in general, I recommend avoiding the powder. For most animals you can just open the capsules and measure out the amount needed. Many dogs will eat the BLM in their food, however in picky dogs keeping the supplement inside a capsule and "pilling" it may be necessary. Although the following doses do not reach toxic levels, by using the capsules, a larger dose can be used as needed, without concern. I generally do not use this supplement in cats due to taste.

- One Capsule = ¼ teaspoon. So for some people, opening many capsules at once, and then measuring out a dose, is much easier.

- Small Dogs – 1/8 to ¼ of a capsule 2-3 times a day.
- Medium Dogs – ¼ - ¾ of a capsule 2-3 times a day.
- Large Dogs – 1 capsule 2-3 times a day.

- Double or Triple the dose if injured acutely, or for the first 6 weeks of administering.

Detoxzyme:

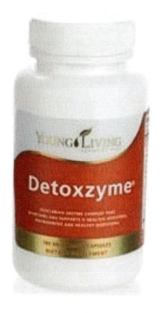

- 1-5 per day depending on severity of the condition, and size of the animal. Generally start with a small amount, and gradually increase.

Digest + Cleanse:

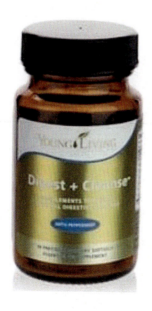

- 1-3 capsules per day – depending on size of the animal and the severity of condition. I generally do not use this supplement in cats.

Inner Defense:

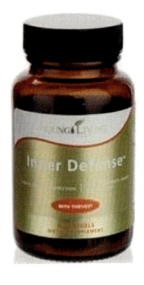

- Cats – generally not used.
- Dogs – dosage depends on the dog and the situation. Inner Defense can disturb gut flora with high doses. When using, give a Life 5 probiotic, generally at night. Make sure that the Life 5 is given 1 ½ to 2 hours apart from the Inner Defense.
- One capsule of Inner Defense contains about 2-3 drops of Oregano, 2-3 drops of Thyme, and 2 drops of Thieves Essential Oil. When needed, homemade capsules can be created.

- Small Dog – starting point 1 capsule.
- Medium Dog – 1-2 capsules.
- Large Dog – 1-3 capsules per day, split into multiple doses.

- In a Large Dog with severe infection, we may even use up to 6 capsules per day.

Juva Cleanse:

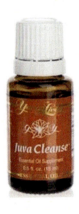

- Cat/Small Dog: 6 drops per day, spread out through the day orally or in a capsule

- Medium Dog: 6-8 drops per day

- Large Dog: 10-12 drops per day

- X-Large Dog: Similar to human dosage – 20 drops per day

K & B Tincture:

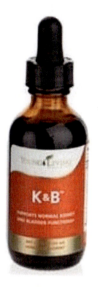

- A small amount more frequently is best. The flavor is not often "appreciated".

- Cats/Small Dogs – a few drops to 1 dropper full multiple times throughout the day.

- Medium Dogs – 1-2 droppers multiple times a day.

- Large Dogs - 3 droppers, three times a day.

Life 5:

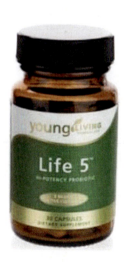

- Keep refrigerated. Give 2 hours apart from oral oils or antibiotics.
- Cats – ¼ of a capsule once or twice a day.
- Small Dogs – ½ capsule once per day, given every 1-3 days.
- Medium Dogs – ¾ - 1 capsule one per day, twice a week
- Large Dogs– 1 capsule per day.
- With severe yeast infections or diarrhea, we may increase the dosage. (Large dogs: 1 capsule 2-3 times a day!)

Longevity:

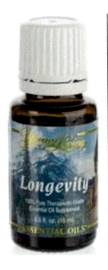 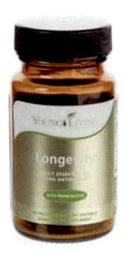

- Helps to keep bugs off animals! It has been noticed that animals ingesting Longevity daily are less "appetizing" to insects.

- Each gel capsule contains about 3 drops of the Longevity Oil Blend.

- Generally not used in cats.

- My dogs will just eat the oil mixed into their moistened food.

- Small Dog – 1 cap per day; or 2-3 drops in mouth per day.
- Medium Dog - 3-5 drops per day.
- Large Dog – 6-7 drops maximum per day.

- Cows – 3-4 drops twice a day, in hay or feed.
- Horses – 3-4 drops twice a day, in lip or feed/supplements.

Omega Blue:

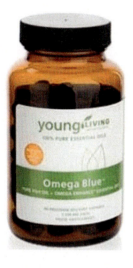

- Cats – I generally avoid these in cats due to size and taste. Some have popped a capsule and tried a drop or two orally, with varying acceptance. Others have given one capsule every 2-3 days. I tend to pick a more "cat friendly" omega fatty acid (such as Standard Process Tuna Omega-3 Oil).
- Small dogs - 1 per day.
- Medium dogs - 2 per day.
- Large dogs - 2-4 per day.

ParaFree:

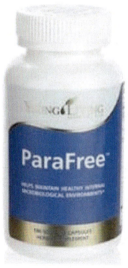

- Cats – Generally do not take this supplement easily. Some have popped a capsule and squeezed a small amount directly in the mouth. An alternative for cats is a combination of Ocotea and Copaiba essential oils. Giving up to 3 drops of each oil, twice a week. These can be dripped directly in the mouth (usually with much protest), or placed into a smaller gel capsule which can be found in pharmacies or health food stores.
- For Heartworm Prevention, the following doses have been recommended twice a week:
    - Small Dog – ½ to full capsule.
    - Medium Dog – 1 full capsule.
    - Large Dog - 1 capsule 2-3 times a day.

PD 80/20:

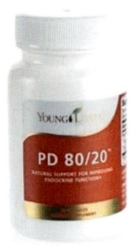

- PD 80/20 is a powerful anti-inflammatory. It contains Pregnenolone, which is a precursor hormone, from which all other hormones are created.
- It is indicated for autoimmune conditions, arthritis, nerve degeneration, and cognitive dysfunction
- Read the Pregnenolone book for more information. You can purchase this book at www.AbundantHealth4u.com.

- Cat/Very Small Dog: A small pinch from an opened capsule per day.
- Small Dogs: ¼ - ½ capsule once a day.
- Medium Dogs: ½ to ¾ capsule per day.
- Large Dogs: Up to 1 capsule per day.
- Give once a day for acute conditions, may be able to maintain on every other day after that.

Rehemogen:

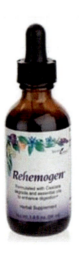

- Blood purifier and builder.
- Cats/Small Dogs: Give 1 dropper per day, until ¼ - ½ of a bottle is given.
- Medium Dogs: Give 1 dropper per day, until ¾ of a bottle is given.
- Large Dogs: Give 1 dropper per day, until 1 bottle is given.
- X-Large Dogs: Give 1-2 droppers per day, until 1-2 bottles are given.

Sulfurzyme:

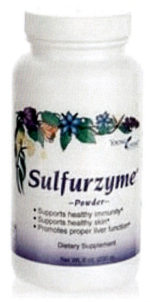

- Thankfully it is almost impossible to give too much of this supplement. If too much is given, soft stools are often noted, and less should be given.
- I usually start with a lower dose, and slowly increase the amount given.
- Sulfurzyme has very little taste, and I find that I can open a capsule, and easily sprinkle the powder onto or into food for any species. The powder can also be used. One capsule contains ¼ teaspoon of powder.
- Great for arthritis, scar tissue, healing...
    - Birds and Exotics – approximately ¼ to ½ capsule per day.
    - Cats – ¼ to 1 capsule per day.
    - Small Dogs – 1 capsule once or twice a day, and up to 1 ½ teaspoons per day.
    - Medium Dogs – 1 capsule twice a day, and up to 1 heaping teaspoon per day.
    - Large Dogs – 2 capsules twice a day, and up to 1 heaping tablespoon per day.

NingXia Red:

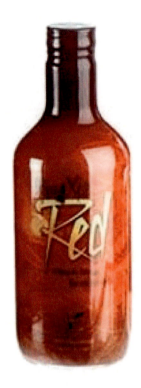

BIRDS & EXOTICS:
- <u>Maintenance</u> – Starting point ½ teaspoon per day.
- I have noticed that some birds and exotic pets seem to require and desire a lot more NingXia Red than most animals. In general, I allow them to "get their fill" – however making sure that they gradually increase their intake as to not get diarrhea or feel ill from the sudden food change.
- <u>Injury or Illness</u> - In severe illness, I may allow them to drink as much as possible without restriction. For example, we had a ferret patient who was diagnosed with Lymphatic Cancer. He was not doing well, and his veterinarian said he would be dead by morning. He had an incredible desire to drink the NingXia Red and would not eat or drink anything else. He consumed several ounces of NingXia Red per day, and continued to improve every day!

CATS:

- <u>Maintenance</u> - ½ teaspoon per day.
- <u>Injury or Illness</u> – up to 1 Tablespoon twice a day or more.

- The sicker they are, the more NingXia Red you should give. Even up to several ounces per day. Best to be given in small frequent amounts.
- Some cats completely hate NingXia Red and some cats devour it. Try it plain, diluted in water, mixed with canned food, or any other crafty way – to get your feline to eat or drink it.
- In cats that completely refuse or have an incredible aversion to the NingXia Red (foaming at the mouth, etc...) I will simply just choose not to give it to them.

DOGS:

- <u>Maintenance</u> –
    Small Dogs: ¼ ounce per day
        Medium Dogs: ½ ounce per day

    Large Dogs: ¾ ounce per day

    X-Large Dogs: 1 ounce per day
- <u>Injury or Illness</u> - Double to Triple amounts – and even more for severe illness. Dividing up amounts and giving it several times a day is best.

HORSES:

- Add to hay or oats, add to water, or syringe
- <u>Maintenance</u> – 1-2 ounces per day – start slowly and build up
- <u>Performance</u> – 3 ounces per day
- <u>Injury or Illness</u> – 4 ounces per day

Whole Food Supplements
What are they, and why do we need them?

All commercial pet food (and most human food for that matter) is processed, cooked, and extruded these days. This process destroys nutrients contained within the food. Most of us have been taught that eating a raw vegetable is healthier for you than a cooked or canned vegetable. When ingredients are added to pet food prior to making it into kibble, the pet food companies know that nutrients will be destroyed in the cooking process, so after the kibble is made – they spray more vitamins and minerals back onto the food. By doing this, if the regulatory companies were to check the guaranteed level of nutrients contained in the food – the levels would still be adequate.

This sprayed on "nutrient liquid" is composed of laboratory created synthetic vitamins. In nature, vitamins exist in complexes. Vitamin C has approximately 5 components to it. I say approximately, because as science discovers "new" vitamin complexes – the fact is that these vitamin components have been there the entire time – contained within REAL FOOD. We just hadn't discovered them yet. If you eat an orange or other Vitamin C containing food – you will get the entire Vitamin C complex – whether we have named a certain complex or not. If you consume Vitamin C that is provided to you through a synthetically created vitamin supplement – you are limited to what a laboratory has created and what science has said is important for you to have. Unfortunately, even quality "natural" vitamin supplements are usually laboratory derived.

Do you remember a few years back, when all of a sudden Lutein became an important nutrient, and was "discovered" to be so good for so many things? I remember hearing vitamin commercials, "Brand X, NOW WITH LUTEIN...." Well, where was Lutein before it had a name? It was still in all natural, real whole foods. It just wasn't in any commercial vitamin. The interesting fact is that Standard Process has had a human supplement called Catalyn since 1929. Catalyn would be similar to what your multi-vitamin is trying to emulate, just in a whole food version. Shockingly, every time a "new" vitamin is discovered, Catalyn has been analyzed and found to already contain that "new" nutrient!!!

This similarity is shockingly similar to essential oil quality. Having the entire complex that Nature intended, is incredibly important to our health, healing, and avoidance of "side effects". This fact is abundantly clear whether you are talking about an essential oil or a whole food.

What happens when we don't receive the entire vitamin complex from a supplement? Unfortunately, nature's master plan is the conservation of what is normal or natural. Vitamin C wants to exist in a full and complete complex. When we take massive doses of only 1 or 2 of these synthetic parts, our body (and nature) wants to complete the complex. So, we will leach the other components out of our bones, muscles, blood etc... to form a complete complex. This process essentially robs our body of the other parts of the complex, causing deficiencies and potential illness. The sad truth is, many of the vitamins that we are taking in an effort to get healthy and stay healthy, may actually be making us sicker.

Why can't we just get our nutrients from the foods we eat? Let's be honest here. Even people I meet (myself included) who eat mostly organic foods, and try to eat a balanced and healthful menu – do not have ideal diets. Add to this the fact that foods today do not even contain the same amount of vitamins, minerals or enzymes that they did 40 years ago. Our soils are depleted. Food is harvested before it is ripe. Even organic produce is shipped over thousands of miles to reach our plates. You can tell the distinct difference by comparing a vine ripened tomato grown in your own backyard, to a store bought tomato (even organic). There is just no comparison. A tomato ripened the way nature intended is still accumulating vitamins, minerals and enzymes as it is "connected to the plant and the earth". There is no substitute for this.

If you think about the majority of pets today – very few of them get any fresh foods at all. The pet food industry has done a great job brain washing us to believe that offering "people foods" to our pets will be detrimental to their health! Quite honestly, if you are eating junk – then yes, table scraps are junk. But, if you offer your pets table scraps of good wholesome foods – then they are probably better off than with commercial pet foods alone!

Pets and humans are just becoming more and more vitamin deficient with each passing generation. I believe that most animals (this includes humans) are actually *born* deficient now. Especially with puppy mills and rescued pets, animals are starting out life, born to a malnourished mother. Then the cycle continues to worsen as we feed them commercial pet foods, with synthetic and non-complete vitamin complexes. Even in the best situation with top quality pet foods – the amount of nutrition to create a healthy litter and then nurse them to weaning; depletes the mother further of any extra vitamins, minerals and enzymes she had to spare.

Part of the theory of feeding pets raw diets addresses this problem. Raw whole foods contain natural and whole vitamin complexes, minerals and natural enzymes. However, since our foods do not contain ideal levels of nutrients any longer, we cannot rely on raw diets alone to fix this problem. I often see pets on a raw diet, who are getting a human multi-vitamin to "complete their nutrition". Not only is this synthetic vitamin a problem as stated above – but I have noticed a trend that some raw feeders, will pick the cheapest generic human multi-vitamin to supplement with. Kind of defeats the purpose of the diet! I strongly feel that even with quality raw diets, all pets need an addition of a truly complete, raw, and "unprocessed" whole food supplement.

Standard Process has a unique and patented technique designed to cold process foods to maintain all of the raw, natural nutrition and enzymes contained within the foods. All of the plant materials used in Standard Process supplements are organic. They have a 1000 acre farm in Wisconsin where they grow and process all of their ingredients – from Seed to Supplement. The food supplements also contain "glandulars". Glandulars are organs and "other parts" of cows, sheep, pigs, etc… Glandulars are an important part of nutrition for pets, as in the "wild" they would be eating hearts, kidneys, intestines, brains, even skin, tendons, and bone. Almost the entire carcass would be consumed by a predatory species. Although the company is working towards being 100% organic – there are not enough organic glandular materials available currently to supply this need. So, glandulars contained within the supplements are not organic.

At this time, I feel that it is far more important for these nutrients to be within the product than that they be organic. Glandulars are extremely important in that they contain nutrients specific for that organ or tissue system. For example, if you eat nutrients that are good for your liver – they will "go" to your liver. Any extra nutrients your liver does not need at the time, will be stored there for future use. So, if you turn this concept around – when you EAT liver it is good for your liver. If you eat skin (yuck) – it is good for your skin. Eat bone, and it is good for your bone. We used to do this all the time in our country – but we have unfortunately come to rely on only parts and pieces of the animals that we sacrifice in the name of food. In the "olden days", we consumed thick stocks made from boiled bones and cartilage. We ate tongue, heart, brain, kidneys, thymus (sweet breads), and other glandulars. Culturally, this has fallen out of favor. However, I am sure your dog or cat would not discriminate given the choice.

Basic nutrition is obviously necessary for daily life and function. But, nutrition is *incredibly* important in healing. Chronic ear infections, skin infections, surgical incisions etc... cannot heal without good nutrition. This is a proven medical fact, and is extremely supported by traditional medical research (even if the medical doctors and veterinarians don't realize it). When recurrent problems continue to crop up after medications have been stopped – this is a clear indication that the body does not have all of the tools necessary to heal itself. Medications are not meant to HEAL anything. Medications are meant to suppress a problem long enough for the body to catch up and heal itself. This is an important concept to understand.

Why not only use Young Living supplements for pets? Don't get me wrong, I think Young Living supplements are second to none! However, they were formulated for humans – and are vegetarian based. Although they can provide some amazing nutritional benefits to cats and dogs, they will never complete the full nutritional picture for an obligate carnivore such as a cat.

I currently only recommend Standard Process Supplements, as I feel they have the quality and results that I see within Young Living Essential Oils. They are the supplements that I consistently see astonishing results with. Several patients had improvements of 75-100% in chronic, recurrent conditions once an appropriate whole food supplement was added into their previous regime. When I combine advanced nutritional support with essential oils, the results are no less than *miraculous*.

You can learn more about this company on their website: www.StandardProcess.com. Products are only available through veterinarians and other health care professionals. You can order the entire line of human and veterinary supplements, as well as the herbal supplements through our veterinary hospital. Just contact us through our website or via email for more information. www.CrowRiverAnimalHospital.com or CrowRiverAnimalHospital@gmail.com.

Thank you for purchasing this book, I sincerely hope that it helps you in your quest for natural animal care.

You can find more information about Dr. Melissa Shelton and educational opportunities, books, webinars, and classes at www.OilyVet.com.

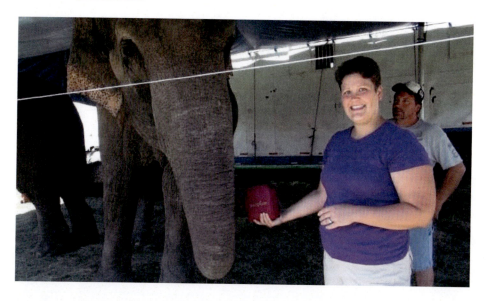

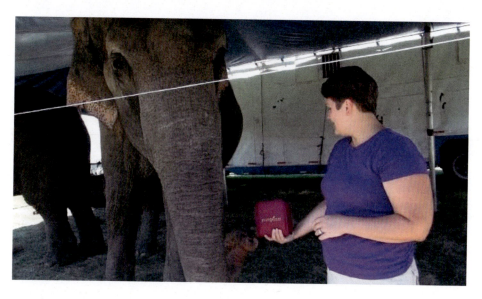

Made in the USA
San Bernardino, CA
22 November 2017